AWAKEN MOVEMENT:
The Key to Life

~

The Body's Way of Knowing

Josef DellaGrotte

Core Integration Training Institute, Inc.
PO Box 95
Barre, MA 01005
Office: (978) 461-0221
www.dellagrotte-somatic.com

Acknowledgments

So many hands have contributed to this book in one form or another. Staying on track was the greatest challenge. There have been several supporters too numerous to mention in this endeavor to move beyond the approaching last stages of the conventional and the current crises into a creative paradigm shift. They certainly include those teachers ancient to modern, from Siddhartha Gautama the Buddha, the Zen Buddhist and Tibetan masters of the science and art of being, the Indian teacher Osho, The Taoist practices of Mantak Chia, to Moshe Feldenkrais and Ida Rolf. Further inspiration came from the *somatic*-field breakthrough books of John Ratey Daniel Coyle, Henry Lodge and Norman Doidge. Then there are all my *Core Movement Integration* colleagues, now teachers and trainers especially in The United States and Italy who have made contributions and continue developing this emerging but not yet publically understood endeavor, and whose names can be found on the respective websites.

www.dellagrotte-somatic.com

www.coreintegration.it

Editing and design production all the way to publication was in the hands of Dina Polizzi who patiently guided me through many rewrites.

The support from professional published authors and friends such as Paul Davidovits, Ph.D. and Ronald Leifer, MD, made the difficult easier.

Note to the Reader

Instructions From Within: Six Pathways to Lifelong Fitness and Wellness, my first book, described the body's core pathways in graphic detail and provided illustrated lesson-exercises which the reader could then visually follow and perform with accompanying text guiding steps. This earlier book covered a wide range of perspectives, cognitive, somatic and instructional .

This second book is about revealing and describing the bigger picture: how to see and read the times and the signs and then to enter into, fully explore and describe the biological, biomechanical and neuro-myofascial sources, structures, and networks that the body-brain generates and signals to us, stimulating not only good but conscious movement and continuing improvement throughout our lives. This all leads to the necessity of walking the talk, listening and recognize body-brain instructions, decode them, map the course, choose the program that works, and jump in!

www. dellagrotte-somatic.com

www.core-integration.com

Contents

Foreword

For the past 40 years Josef DellaGrotte has been one of my most influential and effective teachers. This book provides an entry into the uniqueness and power of his teachings. Josef started his career as an historian.

The early 20ᵗʰ century Spanish-American philosopher George Santayana coined the aphorism "Those who cannot remember the past are condemned to repeat it." However, observations make it evident that even those who do remember the past, learn very little from it. Steeped in the events of the 1960's Josef soon realized that history did not provide answers to the dilemmas and predicaments of modern life. He resigned his tenured university appointment and began to explore alternate paths.

He undertook intensive studies in a variety of modalities, Eastern and Western, becoming well-versed in them both as a practitioner and as a teacher. In the early 1970's he encountered the teachings of Moshe Feldenkrais and began to study this method of body work. He found the work, teachings and scientific logic of Feldenkrais most compelling, enrolled in the first USA Feldenkrais training program, and a few years later Josef started to teach Feldenkrais courses in the Boston area. It was at this point in my early forties that I met him, and was in the grip of a constant and severe backache that at this point had almost completely taken over my life. I attended one of Josef's presentations on the Feldenkrais approach which made immediate sense to me, then enrolled in his course. After many months of classes, slowly I began to gain a sense of my body and its organization. My backache gradually remitted and finally I was pain free. After years of useless medical consultations and interventions, this process of healing seemed almost miraculous. I continued to study with Josef and very clearly my coordination and physical abilities continued to improve.

Josef himself continued to learn. He had studied physical therapy, and Ida Rolf's structural integration method, experimented with myofascial mapping and release techniques, energy flow and a variety of meditation practices. At each stage Josef brought these new learnings into his work and teaching. Over the years his growing insights and skills kept his teachings alive, vibrant and evolving.

Perhaps his most impressive contribution has been his original insights into the Feldenkrais method itself. It has long been evident to many of us who have studied and worked with this technique that the process lacked a clear system of teaching the method and a logical approach to applying it. To become proficient in the Feldenkrais method required literally years and years of trial and error procedures that discouraged many from staying with the training and acquiring the proficiency to help themselves and others with this potentially powerful instrument.

After years of experimentation Josef achieved a remarkable simplification of the Feldenkrais process. He deconstructed the hundreds of Feldenkrais exercises into six basic body movement directional pathways now called *Core Movement Integration*. The system is still not trivially easy. Proficiency and useful integration of the movements requires patience and perseverance. But the process now has a systematic description of a map that allows a much more available access to healthy functional movement.

The technique is well described in available videos, articles and this book. Classes continue to be taught by Josef and his trained teachers. Many hundreds of people have benefited from Josef's teachings. Their movements have improved and they regained often long lost mobility. With patience and perseverance, I am certain that you will likewise benefit.

Paul Davidovits
Professor of Chemistry, Boston College
Author of *Physics in Biology and Medicine*

September 17, 2016

Introduction
Asleep or Just Confused:
No Map, No Plan

How many of us grew up believing that good health, flexibility, self confidence, feeling able, well and fit for a good long lifetime run was either to be expected or supported as a reward for good moral behavior? Is it just a matter of chance and good fortune for those naturally selected out and so blessed, or something requiring too much effort and therefore only for the young, the genetically endowed?

So what happens when the bubble bursts? You start to notice increasing body disorders, inescapable viral infections, discomfort and pain. You are told by your physician, "It's just normal aging, arthritis, or genetics causing you all these problems." Whatever the condition - heart, high blood pressure, diabetes, and the rest of the current top ten nation wide disorders - doctors assure, "We can treat you." No doubt that this is a gentler way to go out than waiting for and enduring the worst. If you are now among the minority who have made it through your middle years without chronic pains, stiffness, and other physical disorders - consider yourself fortunate. Don't keep hoping it will continue by doing nothing!

The mindset of assumed unavoidable degeneration in getting older was a given, and still is. The consequence? Sooner or later when the body starts having problems, we somehow get hypnotically trance-induced to accept this as inevitable. What might follow is some form of medical explanation sounding scientific. Enter the "white coats," the new socially sanctioned and empowered authorities who give some approximation of a diagnosis that looks scientific, and many times is not always so. They prescribe medications, pain pills, a panoply of ongoing tests, corrective surgeries, and other continuing therapeutic interventions to keep us going. Some people who do not find answers with the medical establishment get desperate, try a variety of alternatives, some helpful, some more woo-woo esoteric, and may even turn to forced vigorous exercise to ward off the dreaded *"gombo"* of impending body decline. Is this the path to a better life, or can it also intensify more fear-based stress, worry, and insecurity? How we give our own inner healing power away is a story in itself!

Everywhere I go, here and abroad, person to person, the story is the same: getting older, having more problems, with the bigger closeted problem looming large - aging parents or close relatives who require enormous amounts of extended nursing or home care. Every 4 seconds there is another case of Alzheimer's in the Western world, a documented crisis if not turned around. How long can this go on? It has been possible so far only because of the patrimony, the investments and savings, plus most important, a partially protective government insurance social net (Medicare, Medicaid) that can help you pay for all these services. Unless there is a major upswing in economic growth, an upsurge not yet on the distant horizon, it will be impossible to sustain the amount it takes to keep people going. Some are predicting the increasing debilitations, and especially the super draining costs of dementia, unless halted, will break the economic bank. Yet this crisis can be turned around. That is what this book is all about. And it will have to begin with this generation, as early as possible.

The big picture, the studies and the trajectories surrounding our present state of self-help and health may look more discouraging than optimistic, with no visible changes forthcoming on the health horizon. On the other side, for the first time we have the knowledge and science available to not only maintain a level of wellness for years longer, but also be excited about enhancing that elusive *quality of life* which enables us to continue to do activities that are meaningful and satisfying throughout our life span. And then, the big missing piece: how to make it a reality, not just another set of expectations, not another unrealistic "pie in the sky" about what might change the direction of the current descent. Between these two polarities a new synthesis is arising out of biological foundations with science backing it. Yes, there are obstacles along this path. They need to be identified and addressed. We all sense, but cannot identify, what it is that seems off the track.

From our early optimistic years to our middle and later years, what many people are sensing but cannot get a coherent picture about, is a noticeable disconnect within our own body perception. Most other creatures seem to have a connection with the bio-physical ground of being. They know how to move and do it well. On the human side, and demonstrably shown to be related with our life style, something seems to have gone wrong in the way we are treating our body - all components included.

Simply observe the way people move, the shuffling gait, curved backs, and poor postures. Observe also the prevalence of pain syndromes, dependency on treatment, medications, surgical interventions. What looks normal is actually a sign of slow degeneration. Not a good trend at all. The good news is that the body can relearn, return, re-enter the biological sphere of natural intelligence and intuition, the way to wellness and fitness, and at almost any reasonable age. *We now know that aging is not about getting worse, but can be a biological period in which we certainly slow down, but also get better and wiser at self-management.* We can reduce the negative effects of what has in recent times come to be expected, namely body-mind decline, and actually improve in some important areas of everyday functional life.

If all this has meaning and interest for you, now not later is the time to improve your quality of life, explore new territory, let go of old notions and beliefs about movement and exercise, and increase your longevity/wellness potential, then read on.

One thing is guaranteed - this real inner journey is not a head trip, but rather leads toward a process best designed to shift your orientation, upgrade your internal GPS navigational skills, and lead you into those promised greener pastures only written about, shown in films, and seldom actualized in real life experience. This is the kind of functionally enhanced and healthful living we are capable of, but poorly prepared for.

These landscaping tools will allow you to rediscover, regrow, and revitalize your basic foundation. Being in a human biological body we are subject to the laws of nature - especially gravity and physiology - and clearly more psychologically grounded and secure when we can do activities we prefer, choose, and enjoy. This I'll refer to as our daily life functional movement potential. When we are in this basic zone, common to all creatures large or small, we feel, think, act better, and make more of the right choices. In effect we live longer and well with a good chance of an extended run and closing - like the elephants and other animals who walk until their last day! Most would choose, with just few exceptions, to enjoy each day (*carpe diem*) and experience true quality of life (*qualita di vita!*) To be fully enabled in the here and now we can safely assume is a highly desirable state. With this foundation we can, as will be shown, stay well even with aging. The key, as with any good investment seeking greater return, is to start early.

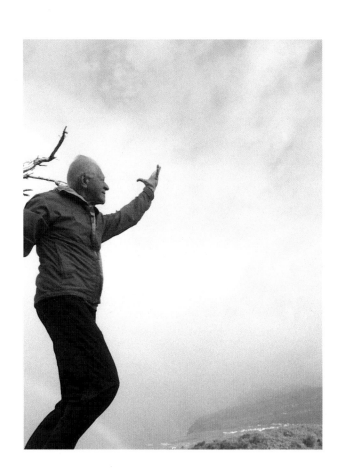

Chapter 1
How I Began My Journey of Discoveries

Gautama the Buddha was once asked,
"Who are you?"

He responded, "I am awake."

"Well, what does that mean?"

"I show a way out of suffering and how to live a more wholesome life."

A few words from an old source of wisdom struck me so many years ago, and remain with me like an echo:

"I have set before you today life and good,
death and evil."[Deuteronomy]

From its roots in the Old Testament theological story to the Buddha and beyond, right to the present day, what does this really mean? What I took away was a simple straightforward message, which could have come from any number of perennial wisdom sources: *Living well or dying badly, you choose!*

Later on, informed by the new emerging knowledge about how the brain-mind functions, one meaning succinctly stated is this: *Without intention, mapping, action and direction, nothing changes.* Add into the mix another elusive but sound observation gleaned from several sources and neuro-psychology: *You cannot say yes and no at the same time!*

Our brain-nervous systems do not work that way. It would be very confusing to any creature to give two simultaneous ambivalent signals, especially if there were emotional charges behind them. Which way to act, react, respond? In real-life situations this would be described as self-conflict. Okay, so do not feed the habit or tendency to be in self-conflict or ambivalence, because whatever you feed will grow.

Moving on to another discovery of neuroscience: "*The brain that fires together wires together.*" Again, what does it mean in terms of living, moving, breathing, learning, habits, illness, pain, health and well-being? We know that the brain and all its body-working components can create and seems to prefer wiring patterns of action and behavior that are functionally satisfying, health promoting, and conducive to generating a sense of well-being. Conversely, the same firing/wiring can go wrong, creating an increase in body disorders and diseases in people stressed out both physically and mentally. It turns out then that this can be either a blessing or a curse! Wired up to be in self-conflict and dysfunctional, it becomes a curse (more pains and suffering); wired up closer to the body's natural, instructional design, the biological imperative, it becomes a blessing (health, well-being). And so full circle we move!

A Journey Through Time

My path of personal growth, discovery and changes in intention and direction came into first flowering in the 1960's. It was one of those unforgettable neo-renaissance like times when change was in the air. With the influx of new arrivals from the East (mind-body practices from yoga to meditation), and the perception altering, mood changing, body-experiencing chemical-psycho ingestants, change was for many the momentum order of the day. The problem was having no clear map or direction except to go with the flow. For me the times were exciting, promising, and near visionary, both as a student in college, then onto grad school. I emerged as a proto-psychedelic East-West version of a reborn seeker/avatar, disguised in that safe and secure mantle of a university professor.

My more interesting colleagues were integrative thinkers. *Interdisciplinary* was the new designation. The beginning of a movement that would take some academics, once safe in the familiar castle, out of the closed box of their own fields and specialization into different ways of thinking and perceiving. My curiosity to cross boundaries took precedence, so I crossed over into relatively unchartered territory. I followed paths that brought me into contact with the emerging new age, leading-edge thinkers and explorers who were also bridging fields of knowledge still kept separate by habit and tradition.

The theme in these inner circles was the interconnection of all those separated and categorized fields of knowledge. We sought to integrate. The means to do so were often elusive and challenging. We were after a modern science of being human. We looked to *systems thinking* approaches. While some were now more open to these approaches, others viewed them with distrust. The universities, the professions of psychology - and even to some far lesser extent medicine, rehabilitation, and physical therapy - were experiencing the challenge of change, but still without a clear model or vision.

In that yet to be awakened personal somato-sphere, something was shifting. I was doing apparently fine well into my thirties - jogging, hiking, swimming, playing handball, tennis - until I started having occasional pains in my left hip. An x-ray and brief consult with an orthopedic physician indicated some kind of irregularity (never explained) and that I should at least stop the jogging. As no definitive reason was given I did not heed.

I was introduced to *hatha yoga* in 1968 by a teaching colleague, an historian whose wife discovered yoga to be more interesting and rewarding than the mental, body disconnected world of academic discourse. She had left university life and switched over to teaching privately. At that time yoga was still new. Considered esoteric but with a rich tradition, it represented both an internal feature (going within, relaxing) and an external one (moving one's body in a slowed down, stretch-concentrated way). It offered an increasingly attractive mode of body-mind conditioning. This slowing down movement into meditative mode was changing my somatic self-perception as well. An internal personal paradigm shift had begun, like discovering another quantum psychophysical universe.

Soon after I was introduced to yet another form of integrative holistic practice known as *tai chi qigong*. Chinese in origin, based on principles of the body-mind-spirit connection, it derives from the Taoist tradition of observing and adhering to nature and its principles, particularly body energy movement flow so evident in the animal world. It had even begun to slowly penetrate the thick walls of mind-centered academia! One of my colleagues, a woman in the university's art department, was teaching it on the side. We met. I joined her class. The underground railroad in the university castle was slowly coming alive.

Then came a major breakthrough! Encouraged by a colleague in the business school at the University of South Florida, I applied to do a practitioner training with Ida Rolf (a biologist and founder of an alternative New Age system called *Rolfing*) to be conducted at Pigeon Key in Florida. I managed to get a six-week leave from teaching assignments to attend this special training. Off I went with a few others of similar new age disposition in my area including a psychiatrist and a psychologist. The training opened new doors of somatic perception, another realm radically different from the intellectual academic model mindset. This new form of body-centered rethinking addressed muscle and tissue as the pathways to awaken consciousness

4

in all sectors - physical, emotional and mental. Ida Rolf had created a system designed to restore body function through what was called *structural integration*, a method involving ten intensive one-on-one sessions addressing the newly discovered territory - the body's connective tissue network. This psychophysical approach allowed and even stimulated emotional release in many. The theory was that emotional hang-ups are held in body tissue, and that through physical manipulation release of all kinds might occur, revealing what had long been blocked. The assumption and the attraction of the method was that through the physical all problems could be brought to the surface and hopefully reintegrated.

Ida Rolf was attempting to put together a formularized body-work somatic strategy that she claimed would restore the body to its natural "structurally integrated" condition before corruption from all the negative influences. The process also claimed to break up habitual mental-emotional self-images. This new modality offered a body-mind treatment therapy that was more structured and body-centered, but not contrary to the then *scream it, shout it, act it out, force it out* techniques for physical-emotional release like bioenergetics, primal scream therapy and Gestalt that were capturing public attention. Rolfing involved more forceful bodywork applications, effective when done skillfully, but lacking in listening-in to the more subliminal signals of the body. For someone like myself, an intellectual interested in pursuing just how far the integrative and interdisciplinary model could be developed, the training seminar was yet another world of openings.

During the training Ida would mention others she admired. One in particular was Moshe Feldenkrais from Israel, a well-respected scientist- engineer, graduate of the Sorbonne, and a former associate of Frederick Joliot Curie of the Marie Curie Institute in France. He was turned by life's challenging lessons into a displaced conventional - a career change- shifter transitioning from engineering into somatic practitioner and pioneer.

Feldenkrais had developed a new method that was not easy to understand but yielded results unobtainable in the conventional therapeutic world. He further confounded his conventional supporters by claiming he was "not doing therapy" but only helping people to restore and further develop their body-mind potential through the real education of self-learning. With his science trained perception and out of the box life experiences, Feldenkrais saw that therapy - even the best of proposed treatments - was not enough to overcome the power of habitual body and mind fixations.

Eventually what emerged in the 1970's was his new integrative method to improve not only the growing problems of compromised body and posture but also to redirect human mental-emotional anxiety-driven states to true developmental maturity. The components of the process were called *awareness through movement* and *functional integration*. And who else but such an integrative somatic thinker would, in those times, call his first and successfully published book *Body & Mature Behavior: a Study of Anxiety, Gravitation, Sex, and Learning* (1949)

With no set number of sessions, Feldenkrais's method suggested something radically new, a major departure with a basis in scientific inquiry and process, declaring that there were "no fixed principles," no fixed techniques, no end-gaining results, only how the body learns and changes. The method looked more zen-like with a quasi-professional training process

Moshe Feldenkrais

Moshe Feldenkrais must have been listening to signals from the source within. At age 16 he undertook a journey that would radically change the direction of his life. As he recounted his own life story, he left his Byeloruss-Ukraine village and started walking, at least a good part of the way, some 1000 miles to Italy and then on to Palestine. Fast forward to the late 1930's. As part of a team of well-known scientists in France, he developed the equipment for nuclear fission, and then with the Nazi invasion in 1940 was on the run, a target of the Nazis seeking him out.

that had no preconceived preparation, minimal testing of practitioners and a scarcity of clinical supervision. For many of us its attraction was a breakout from conventionalized textbook learning and public education - something with an eastern approach, but clothed in western garb. It was a good basic integrative combination of physics, evolutionary physiology, biology, psychology and all. Here was a bridge between passive treatment (chiropractic, acupuncture, massage, Rolfing, etc.) to engaged learning.

Feldenkrais was interested in developing the brain using movement awareness as the instrument and the process. By reference to his own journey from science to the somatic arts, he exemplified a way to cross boundaries and integrate the body-mind through movement. Nothing he discovered was entirely new or unknown. The martial arts such as judo and tai chi contain similar principles but are more esoteric. Feldenkrais extracted from them good working applications creating more science based neuro-somatic movement lessons, which could be observed and tested. He re-synthesized and fashioned them into his own method.

I studied with him for nearly a decade. The processes and principles he introduced remain as one of the foundations of my own practice and system of *Core Movement Integration (CMI)*. It is a synthesis of Feldenkrais plus principles from my own training and learning experiences in physical therapy, physics, physiology and myofascial systems, further supplemented with concurrent training in body-centered practices (Gestalt, psychomotor psychology, meditation, yoga, qigong, tai chi, running, upright power walking and hiking).

Many learners settle into a practice, never move much beyond it, and hopefully improve as much as possible within the limiting potentials of the box. My road is different. Something within, that hidden voice, has continuously moved me on to further reaches and developments, always keeping to the path that allows for integration. Along the way I have been occasionally tempted by the sirens of mostly proprietary methods claiming to be the true one - the most valuable and promising. But something within always hesitated to join the "true believers," the ones convinced they have it all or who see only through conditioned inculcated lenses. Even with Feldenkrais, who said he had "no fixed principles" and advocated open inquiry, once post mortem his teachings morphed into the *Feldenkrais Method*®- with proprietary protective trademarks and claiming a purity of the method never defined or agreed upon. The trainings have continued and spread, but have not really grown nor entered the mainstream of alternative modalities. A minority of practitioners have become successful in practice. Others following a universal tendency to discover more have integrated the Feldenkrais principles with other conventional modalities. What is emerging is a seeding effect as new varieties of the original Feldenkrais work are being formed with the same intention: to provide a means of somatic learning that can keep people living well and more self empowered. And I, being similarly inclined, found myself listening more to the observations of such folk as the wise Sufi Omar Khayyam who centuries ago wrote to the effect:

"When I was young I heard great argument about this and that,
from many convinced and strongly bent,
and always left by the same door wherein I went."

My Personal Journey Continued...

Reflecting back to my late thirties, I recall severely and repeatedly spraining my ankle. Hiking and running became problematic. I had to take steps carefully. A pattern of entropy was getting established. Now the new approaches started to kick in.

At that time I was in transition, having decided to leave not only an established career in university teaching, but also planning a shift into rehab counseling and physical therapy. I had decided on

8

the path less traveled. I joined and was well into full certification training with Dr. Moshe Feldenkrais, my feet still in both worlds. By doing new exploratory (non-conventional) movement lessons I was gradually able to stabilize with no further problems.

The next phase came in my early forties when I went off to Nepal to do the long trek leading up to the Solo Kumbu plateau, the direction towards Mt. Everest. Getting ready in Katmandu, my left hip and leg pains started up again. Doing the trek alone there were no doubt psychophysical factors at play. A few months before in India, I had had one of those spiritual crises (arising from my conflicted involvement and forced departure from the Rajneesh Indian ashram) which later I could experience as opportunity for awakenings. I was playing out what I had imagined and internalized from a very charismatic and convincing Indian guru, that I would find my true self through "bliss in aloneness" [Sanskrit: ananda asanga]. But at the start, instead of bliss I was experiencing hip-leg pain recurrence. Hesitant and concerned, I nevertheless decided I would continue, trusting in the body by doing an intense morning preparation using everything I knew, especially the new lesson-exercises I had been learning with Feldenkrais. Doing these different kinds of non-habitual movements significantly decreased the pains, allowing me to walk a little more, get stronger each day and feel more confident.

On about day six my Sherpa guide left claiming illness. By then I was feeling confident, able to continue on my own - reinforced by both the guru's prescription for spiritual *moksha* and now my own manifesting abilities to listen internally and trust the way. I was alone except for occasionally meeting with other so inspired trekkers and seekers during and at the end of the day. I was pain-free and feeling a new level of fitness and endurance, so I continued all the way eventually to the Solo Kumbu, the Kala Patar peak and the base of Mt Everest.

Returning to Katmandu and civilization was both overwhelming and unsettling, so on I went to the Annapurna circuit and after that to Pokara, gateway to the west section of Nepal towards Mustang. I had become a trek rat - increasing my distances and feeling invulnerable. I could truly be alone and blissful. Mission accomplished!

All good things come to an end. I returned home, began running again, and started having some knee and thigh pains. Another foot exam and recommendation to try orthotics which at first worked. Still hooked on the "American way"- that gripping habit of more and faster is better - I decided to upgrade my running form, training with a well-known college coach and new friend to increase speed and distance. Eventually even taught running using different principles in combination with the modified Feldenkrais lesson-exercises I had developed (and being cited in the *Boston Globe* for my new approach).

By then I was a weekend warrior running many local races until one fateful day in Spring 1995 my knee suddenly went out and I could not even walk without pain. An MRI revealed significant tears. Feeling helpless and immobilized and with much hesitation and deliberation I chose arthroscopic surgery (left knee) and watched the procedure. This was the revelation that started me on a new course. I was able to see, follow, map, and reconstruct the lines of force that over the years were shearing the medial meniscus (the most common tear among runners), and had damaged the articular cartilage of the femur, an unexpected additional complication.

This was the time to stop running. I knew by my training as a therapist and movement practitioner that continuing would have guaranteed a knee replacement (many do not stop and later suffer the consequences). I also came to see that walking, not running, would be my path. Born to walk, not run, has always been time-tested and known from way back in human history.

So I gradually took up fast walking, still under that diminished but nevertheless wired-in conditioning, my lifestyle demon, urging *more, faster and longer.* Eventually I took up race walking, at that time a new upcoming niche Olympic sport! It did keep me going for years, changed the angle of force through the knees, a biomechanical alignment,which better protected it. I was on the way to rediscovering how to really walk, approximating what tribal people have always done. Fast walking also satisfied cardio-vascular stimulation and its positive benefits, but still would eventually prove to be another dead end. Continuing to try to keep up speed while getting older is a somatic oxymoron! It doesn't work. The pains began to return. End of competitive race walking!

What to do, where to go next? By now I had developed a new far more evolved set of lesson-exercises in walking, swimming and other activities that have shown to really work and benefit thousands of our clients and students - all using the most efficient alignments from the pelvis through the knees, ankles and feet. This made it possible to walk with few recurrent problems. And so I was inspired in October 2014 to walk the Camino Santiago in Spain with a backpack. During that first trek of 250 miles I experienced knee stiffening and an onset of ankle pain.

On returning I consulted a minimalist orthopedic surgeon, one of the few who deal with both knee and ankle which are structurally connected! The MRI revealed some arthritis, but with no recommended conclusion about what kind of treatment might be needed. The surgeon was skeptical about doing any surgical intervention since it was not clearly indicated. He was one of few in the profession who favored surgery as the last resort. So I was back to listening to signals from within - my inner guide, intuition, leading me again - and devising new movements never done before.

Once more I went into exploratory upgrade mode. First I changed to a recommended better modifiable orthotic, away from the hard, fixed ones I had tried and now rejected. Then I carefully studied how to use foot actions and specific path trajectories, keeping on the *4th metartarsal*, something that Dr. Feldenkrais knew about and had introduced but never fully developed or explained well.

Consulting with only a few colleagues who were open to seeing differently, we began to map track, and cultivate this new but really ancestral approach, now becoming a discernible, definable, anatomically precise pathway. Using our CMI directional mapping system and connecting the foot all the way through to the spine and ribs, we further refined the way to learn and teach this to anyone open to changing habits. It worked!

On my second Camino trek in May 2015, which was 250 more miles in Spain (all the way to Santiago de Compostella and beyond to Finisterre the furthest Camino western point on the European continent) I had only minor occasional inflammations with hip, knee, ankle or foot. I was also able to help several pilgrim trekkers suffering similar problems along the way.

By the third phase in September 2016, continuing on another 200 miles of the French section of the Camino, a new but related

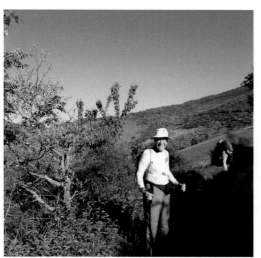

problem in my left hip began to emerge. Catastrophic thought: "Okay the orthopods were right. No escape. Check it out. Get hip replaced if necessary. Showing signs of wear we know. Get with the trend. So many are doing it. You're no exception. After all, parts do wear out…"

Wait, not so hasty, no rush! Again, following what Moshe Feldenkrais and many others had shown, I tried the neuro-somatic relearning approach using the movements I knew. I found relief. Another orthopedist had earlier taken an X-ray of my right side hip joint showing some wear as well, and suggested replacement to support the left side! Good thinking from within the box of routine conventional procedures, but to me not convincing.

Crisis is Opportunity - Meeting the Challenge

My next phase in January 2016 took me to a writing retreat in the mountainous Canary Island of La Palma, with some serious hiking challenges I was not prepared for. Everywhere on the island is either up or down, with a 7000 foot volcano in the middle. After getting myself oriented on some of the more manageable local roadways and trails, feeling more strengthened and confident I decided to try a path that was not on the main trail system. It was indicated only by a number and by occasional white poll markers (from the pueblo of Franceses to Roque del Faro). Starting out, I asked a local goat farmer about this purported marked walking trail. He pointed to a distant sign-post on the road, told me it was marked and that I could not go wrong, it would take me a few hours at most. And so I followed a trail sign indicating 5.8 kilometers. Only thing - it was all up, a 2000 foot climb at a steep angle. The only other way was the less steep 10 kilometers winding main road with cars and such going by. The one thing missing was a likely non-existent map. At Roque there is only one bar-restaurant. So, get some food there and then return by the bus which would come every two hours, or four hours on weekends.

I began the climb on a small road, which turned into a densely vegetated path. I could see the ground beneath me and started to hack my way through, at times without benefit of a machete, which I really needed along with my trekking poles. Every kilometer or so I would find a trail number marker indicating it was still the same.

About 3 km up, a dense fog started coming in. The path eventually came out on the main road, and across was the continuation.

More kilometers through a narrow steep trail, then on to a small country road with no markers, and at a split the choice of which to take. After going left and seeing that it descended into a ravine, I back tracked, took the right - walked almost interminably, came out on another road, and again had to decide to go right or left. Had to guess, and went left. If this did not work out, the thought of going back down the mountain 2000 foot was not an option. Then one car finally came by. I hailed it and they stopped - a Spanish couple on holiday taking this less traveled road with falling rocks and one lane tunnels, on their way to Santa Cruz. They did not know where Roque was - they had passed without noticing this non-descript village. They offered to drive me to Barlovento, some 20km away. I had no choice, I accepted. I had lunch while waiting for the bus back to Franceses on its every 4 hour weekend schedule. I arrived in the dark, trying to grope my way up to my casita on a unlit road with only my footsteps feeling the narrow roadway.

But the failed hike memory, the challenge not completed, kept coming back to haunt me leaving me with unsettling residues. I re-minded myself from some wisdom-system verse that "the only way out is through." I decided to give it a go again and get it right. I also came to realize that these local farmers rarely used these trails, now being habituated to travel by trucks and buses. I would give myself 3 hours or more. This time again following the rainforest vegetation covered trail straight up I came to the main road, did not cross over as before into that other no longer clearly marked path, and decided to go right. I knew Roque had to be still 3-4 km in that direction. After a while I came upon another trail sign indicating a lesser dis-tance. About 15 minutes on the trail the fog increased hiding the overview with more overgrown vegetation. Soon I discovered it was going down steeply, winding on switchbacks into a ravine (bar-ranca) where it would then eventually have to go up again, saving the distance of the winding road but at what additional difficulty or peril? My inner signal instincts kicked in. I stopped, briefly assessed, then turned to go back to the main road. From there I followed it all the way, a little longer and the better decision it turned out to be! I finally arrived at El Roque, had lunch, and caught the last bus back to Franceses.

These walking challenges continued, though less dramatically, on different trails and destinations marked, but involving steep descents and ascents on switchbacks, on near sheer vertical ravines. Sometimes taking the road, sometimes taking the trail. For centuries this is how the pre-public transport islanders made their way. Today only few of the inhabitants use these trails, mostly just the trekker tourists from various European countries.

Finding Solutions

When I returned from the Canaries my left hip was acting up - not a good sign for my next planned Camino trek. Pain, as we will examine, is a signal indicating that something is wrong and needs attention. But the pain does not always reveal the where, how, or why. I remembered that wise lady biologist, Ida Rolf saying, "Where it is, it ain't."

Okay, another challenge, use it to change something! I brought out all my special lesson-exercises and myofascial release techniques, and kept up my walking routine, but the pains continued. Back to the drawing board, I came up with a more precise way of aligning through the hip to direct the forces upwards, unloading and reducing effort on the joints. Yes, I could manage, but this would clearly not keep me going. The pains from going down steep descents for a month on my "goat island" retreat were not abating.

At this point I was convinced I had a slowly developing condition, seen so often in my client practice, called *trochanteric bursitis* (a specific kind of hip pain generated around the femur). It was keeping me awake at night. I began to inquire among my colleagues, getting their views while also applying what I know and self-treating. As usual, almost any kind of treatment may produce some relief for some of the time. By then I had several opinions about it, different perspectives like the blind men and the elephant, helpful intentions much appreciated, but bottom line - was I addressing the root of the symptoms? I challenged my own belief notion of avoidance by deciding to get an X-ray, not only of my left hip but also my right one. Both hip joints are really one system interacting together and affecting each other - an unusual concept in orthopedics given such a specific instance and location of pain.

I chose a very experienced and competent sports doctor (also a distance runner) whom I had searched for and sought out precisely because he did not do hip replacements. He performed a simple but impressive examination testing all angles of motion - no woo-woo, no visual reliance, just real testing of body mechanics 101. The exam was precise, and the findings as close to scientific as one can get. Findings? Not trochanteric at all, but a possible bone spur implication. What followed was cortisone, which failed and resulted in worsening of the condition. And then a recommended MRI revealed "spinal facet compression" with stenosis, but no clear cause-effect. Suggested treatments? Try more cortisone. No surgery indicated. Two cortisone injections later did nothing.

With no further help from the medical profession, and only rising costs, I began to develop a new regime of movement exercises on my own, with help from some like-minded practitioner colleagues - a new launch into the never ending process of either getting better, or eventually getting worse! What has kept me going despite the wear and tear on the joints (specifically the original 1995 knee surgery now also close to "bone-on-bone") is my adaptation, my flexibility and fitness levels. Will my hip joints and spine stay the course? Will they outlast me? Who knows! And even a rare few of those out of the box sports orthopedic doctors and experienced physical therapist colleagues I consulted agree.

Three months later, doing the new mindful core strengthening plus spinal realignment exercises, combined with swimming and a special antigravity treadmill, I was out of pain and back to walking - nowhere near as fast as before, but with much less up-downs. Joints wearing down with both age and many, many miles are evident and undeniable. Not withstanding, the body-brain beat goes on!

The Finale! In July, 2016, I traveled to the Italian Dolomites to conduct a 10 day course on how to walk well and fit, interspersed with several miles of hiking. Lo and behold, my very spine structure had shifted, and I was able to scale these high, well groomed but rugged mountains without any negative repercussions, no problems beyond my age-related wear factors. This now reawakened and inspired a new confidence to return to the Camino Santiago in France, the southern section, and walk another 200 km which I completed in September with no further problems. As the Swiss country people say - and likely the elephants as well - we *walk until the day we die."* I once more know that this shift is possible, but only after we can get out of the medical-therapy dependency cycle, and learn to access the body's signals from within.

Bringing it All Together

No one walks the path of discovery without these antecedents. If they have been embodied they remain a part of you. That is what *integration* is all about, a state in which enough previous experience, perception, skill, application, thinking process, and emotional self-regulation are working together. While incorporating and honoring all that I have previously learned from the rare, true masters of their art and several fine teachers, I found myself moving into further dimensions of *integration* - listening by slowing down to my own intentional voice, instructions from within.

This dimension of my work took me away from the growing community of somatic practitioners settled into comfortable technique-oriented standardized practices onto another level. In this new style of practice, I began to feel more open, creative, better with myself.

This way of practicing offers improved, simplified, easy, clear, and less convoluted and time-consuming applications typical of the modalities in which I had been trained. And the best benefit of all - far less body pains from overworking oneself for lack of both movement skill and awareness.

It is said that you can't solve a problem from within the problem. Personal habits and social habits are interconnected, carrying with them many seeds of hidden somatic disorders plus much unexplained and unwanted suffering. New openings, new perceptions, new experiences and options are becoming available each day. People, recognizing dead ends, are moving towards opening and becoming aware. Supported by the new emerging somatic based sciences, plus the life-style potential benefits, they are slowly discovering how to live well, long and fit until they can then say with no regrets, "goodbye!"

What began with body-mind and movement emerged over time into *Core Movement Integration*, a pathway based program to live well and fit for life. It contains the best of what I have learned and continues to grow and change. *CMI* has very grounding features plus the creativity of working with each individual's specific needs in the context of their body patterns and conditionings. To be successful, to fulfill the intention, everything included in this book just points the way. It is a written form of a mission-vision as a vehicle to communicate both a wake up call and mapping route for those who want to move out of our inescapable entrenched habits.

Chapter 2
Return to The Biological Imperative

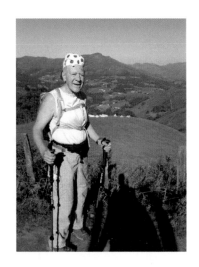

The foundation is already in place. Evolution has done its work. We come into life with a highly developed biological inheritance of precision design and function, a body-brain system that knows what to do, how to move, and works in sync to keep us going well, fit and satisfied enough to want to continue the journey. We have developed the means to extend life — yes, living longer, but not necessarily healthy, well, and fit like most of the creatures on planet earth. To disturb, disrupt, even deactivate some of our basic biological signals takes relearning in the newest part of our big brain, the neo cortex. It happens whenever we stop listening to the habit signals in favor of a different signal source. We are susceptible to superimposed instructions from outside. And so the *biological imperative* can be breached.

Such instances are how we have become dependent on a new authoritative source called medicine. It has been able to do wonders for many. Another is so-called health insurance. Our neo-cortical big brains convince us that providing more treatment is the key to living long and well. It turns out this is not so. By retirement age the percentage of those physiologically and even mentally compromised is higher than sustainable, way off the chart of biological viability and vitality, or economic sustainability. The message is clear: from the known biological perspective, all creatures who have managed to live longer have also learned to live, move, eat well and stay fit, sustained by the body-brain skills to be able to be fully into life and enjoying it!

Either You Are Getting Better or You Are Getting Worse!

That is what marks *the biological imperative.* The first step is to get back on track, tune in to what has always been there and follow the system's path toward improvement. There really is no other choice. The mythic story of heaven was the centuries old answer to a life of pain, stress, disease and suffering. That mythic story no longer works and will not sustain or provide much solace to the many millions going through body-mind degeneration accompanied by greatly limited functional movement, pain and often depression. Simply living longer unprepared stands in stark contrast to the biological imperative. Game over! *Les jeux sont fait!* Continuing to follow the same habits that do not work results in conditioning them deeper, often into chronic pain patterns as we see and now recognize. Some Eastern wisdom teachings call it *samsara,* the realm of suffering.

Signals from the Source: Where to Begin and How

The key to the survival, health and wellness of any species, particularly our own, is in how to access built in signals from within, body intelligence or intuitive knowing. Where do they come from?

Anything alive has some form of DNA coding, some built-in behavioral information and programming. When we humans lived closer to nature the signals came through much more clearly, much like the animals who know how to move, react and respond instantly, how to navigate skillfully, and make decisions moment by moment. Sometimes making mistakes cost! In more developed species this coding can be influenced and modified through experience. Creatures learn new behaviors. How this all gets passed on we will leave to the geneticists to argue about.

The reality from the get-go is that all creatures, ourselves included, have our basic body roots in the biological and biomechanical ordering of nature. We learn to move and develop under the instructions specific to our phylogenetics. We are led into our development without directing it. Our entire DNA guided nervous system responds to the stimuli of life to meet our most basic needs. Here are some essentials to maintain our needs and do our daily, hopefully satisfying activities:

1. Good nutrition
2. Good sensing and moving — expressed in the right kind of exercise, play, and relaxation
3. Nurturance, acceptance, and support

Then onto higher levels — especially human needs like:

4. Care and affection, love
5. Wholesome interactions with others (common good, satisfying to all)
6. Enjoyment, curiosity and creativity
7. A sense of purpose

Having at least the basic needs fulfilled is now universally recognized as an internal stabilizing foundation — settling the wild tendencies of the human central nervous system (the *cns*). Human beings have a higher (and more dangerous) level of fear, anger, and distress, which gets triggered from all forms of perceived basic deprivation of needs. When needs are not met the nervous system generates very unsettling, unpredictable behaviors leading to life-long disturbance, suppressions or acting out without satisfaction— all internalized in the body. *"I can't get no satisfaction!"* So have those astute psychologists and other pioneers of somatic studies observed and demonstrated. These now negatively embodied somatic restrictions can slow down, even arrest, the human biological maturation process. All of this gets held in various sectors of the body-brain complex. Neuroscience is revealing for the first time the body's long held secrets.

Basic needs seem to be a biological imperative, the starting point. How they are met is the challenge, the positive stress of life. The first thing is then how to move well. As Feldenkrais noted, "movement is the key to life."[1] Without this foundation, our attempts to satisfy any higher level needs become insecure and unpredictable. Imagine any structure that has a weak foundation. Everything built on it is less stable.

The next set of needs can now get fired up and wired such as how to take care of oneself; what kind of movement based practical learning to engage in to improve *quality of life*; how to cultivate the essential ingredients to support the body-mind system for life. This will involve making necessary changes and improvements from time to time, usually updating or reprogramming earlier adaptive behaviors that are no longer appropriate, no longer work. But this does not come by mental thinking alone. That often just spins our wheels. The brain can only change by doing, that is by moving in a more efficient and satisfying way. The key is through practice, through interest and the pursuit of self-care—physically, mentally, and emotionally. The concept is as old as mankind, but like love, peace and intelligent choices, not often applied when most needed. No creature can maintain a lasting level of wellness without this foundation and its implementation into a skillful means of living.

---

1 Out of print, still available, not the easiest read but worth it: M.Feldenkrais, **Body and Mature Behavior**, 1949, Harper & Row — a pioneering work in its time. His insights, findings and conclusions have more recently been recognized by medical neuroscientists such as Norman Doidge, MD, and earlier by the body-mind oriented psychologists and somatic practitioners such as Abraham Maslow, Wilhelm Reich, Alexander Lowen, Fritz Perls, Carl Rogers, Roberto Assagioli and now many others. Contemporary neuroscientists such as M. Merzenich, John Ratey,MD, Henry Lodge, MD describe the brain's activity behind this]

Knowing, Thinking and Moving

Pains come and go. They are inevitable. Chronic suffering is optional.

You may have heard the story—real or not – of the frog that was put into its normal water temperature, which then was gradually heated up so gradually that it never jumped out and eventually died. Real or a metaphor it reveals the condition our condition is in.

The French mathematician and philosopher, Renee Descartes [17th century], with his self -proclaimed great discovery "I think therefore I am," is an example of a cultural body-mind-spirit split so characteristic of early modern times. Imagine his long pondered effort to substantiate his existence and coming up with such a conclusion so dissociated from any internal body knowing. Every other being on earth knows itself first through sensing and moving. In spite of his brilliance, Descartes could not really verify the proof of his existence except by his observation that he was thinking! Did he never notice he was eating, drinking, moving, breathing, sitting and walking?

Internal Mapping: Knowing Where You Are, Who You Are

A 12-year-old African boy from a migrant tribe was put in a local school by his parents as his only chance to get an education. By the time the schooling period finished, his family and tribe had already moved on great distances through trackless jungle unmarked by any usual signs. He still manages to find them. How did he do it? Is it just intuitive, or something more? Is the path an image that his central nervous system intelligence can work out? Does the way he and countless others manage to navigate and find their way have anything to do with cues from sensing, moving, and body-centered thinking?

A cat is accidentally left behind by its owners who have returned home, some 200 miles away. Some time later the cat finds its way home. How does the cat or the dog, in many recorded instances, know how to find the way?

The Sufi master, Omar Khayyam, saw through these mental self delusions: (I paraphrase) *"In my day I visited scholars and philosophers, and heard great argument about this and that, and in the end, always left by the same door wherein I went."* [The Rubayyat]

Movement and functional exercise not only stimulate the brain but are fundamentally connected with thinking and intelligence. In the animal brain as in the human, thinking is a body-brain function designed to bring about a result by changing some variable of behavior. Animals can manipulate, or just use their body action skills in ways that accomplish some specific result. This thinking still involves basic level consciousness, but not awareness as we know it. The predator has to figure out the right moves to catch the prey. This is learned conscious behavior. Movements in the right order bring results. Even the prey learns how to maneuver to confuse the predator. These decisive thinking actions make the difference of life or death. The explanation of calling it just instinct is an after the fact conclusion (ex post facto) and explains nothing. Humans can use thinking in a functional way, or in a dysfunctional way. Thinking that does not involve applications in the real setting of here and now is abstract, driven by one's own limited perceptions and often not related to reality. This can create false thinking. What we imagine is the case may not be that way at all. It has to be checked out.

Operational-Organizational Basics: Cars, Boats, Machines and Drivers

Here is a simplified model and approach that almost anyone who drives or operates any moving machinery can understand. You may have a well-made car (boat, airplane, bicycle, machinery, whatever), but if you do not know how to operate it, you can ruin it and injure yourself. Similarly, even if you have a defective system (machine or body), but you know how to use it well and maintain it, you can at least get by. The best option is to have both. That way it all works better and lasts much longer, and you might even enjoy things more! The difference is that the machines we rely on cannot improve themselves. The human body conditioned through evolutionary experience can improve or get worse depending on how it is being used. The only condition that really matters is the neuro-somatic movement programming by which it learns and changes.

This combination of basic biology—being born in a body in whatever genetic condition it may be—and the learning skills we develop and use for whatever our condition may be in tells it all. Depending primarily on instructions from outside sources, good as they may be, is disempowering. By example, reflect on the old Ten Commandments control model dictated from on high, and now the new secular forms: commanding authorities who will not even allow you to walk, like the elephants, to your burial grounds of choice. It is very difficult to make the transition in the way you might choose! Another disadvantage to simply following instructions—not yet clinically verifiable but suspected—is that it may further inhibit self motivation and much needed brain stimulation as we age, generating more neuronal plaque.

Misdirecting natural biological priorities carries with it serious compromises leading to the long slow slippery slope of body-mind disorders, disease and degeneration. Extending life without quality of life is a set up for depression further fueling degeneration. As the Greek philosopher Socrates put it long ago, *"The unexamined life [i.e. without awareness of interconnections] is not much worth the living."*

There may be additional needs required for growth, health and self-development, but without this foundation they risk becoming distorted, confused, compromised, and unable to be truly satisfied. All this is revealed in the body though we may deny, disguise, suppress or cover up. Or as Gautama Siddhartha the Buddha, observed, *suffering begins with ignoring, not wanting to see what is (avidya).*

What is Happening to Us?
How Can We Reverse It?

We are adaptable but only to a certain degree. For example, if we eat too much, or the wrong foods, the consequences will be not only obesity but many new disorders, among them heart diseases, diabetes, and cancer.[2]

When the biological foundation is compromised, a breach in the body's wall of health takes place. Though our food supply is much improved and our medical treatment methods apparently far more developed, we cannot claim that we are much better off. Current evidence and research indicate that postural and joint problems are on the increase. It's not hard to connect the dots. The dramatic decrease in our daily need requirements of movement exercise has already led to a host of new body problems that neither paleolithic nor primitive peoples may have experienced. They did die younger, but this is all relative. You get no reward points now or later for living longer. The real points reward is in living better!

Despite our cerebral stimulation through mass education, our university brain centers, our high-dependency value and emphasis on mental development, we have neglected what now is known as the essential ingredient to a healthy brain and nervous system: **sustained exercising**. Lacking this we have also become susceptible to a new class of brain-deteriorating disorders from dementia to Alzheimers, stroke, and Parkinsons.

Awareness, intention and practice, often considered the foundations of most personal development and spiritual practices, is the heart of what the ancient Chinese sages called the *Tao*, the *Way*. In its fullest sense it is a door between two or more ways of seeing which offers more choices. While the habitual way of doing things may work well, it becomes less functional and less intelligent when

2   One powerful read is Colin Campbell, *The China Study*, a comprehensive research based and statistical analysis of these prevalent debilitating diseases and what they have in common.

26

driven by anxiety. The other choice is intention. Once any human being is interested in opening the door of perception, new options arise. It's simply part of the *way* of living, sensing, moving and feeling internally connected.. The awareness option leads to being able to do what we intend.

Chapter 3
Crisis and Change

"It's a characteristic of human nature that
the best qualities called up quickly in a crisis are
very often the hardest to find in a prosperous calm.
The contours of all our virtues are shaped by adversity"

- Gregory David Roberts, **Shantaram**

Story From History

In the year 1348, the Bubonic Plague known as the "Black Death" struck the European continent and British Isles, eventually wiping out from 25-50 percent of the local populations. The plague spread mostly in populated cities, towns and villages. In the religious mindset of the times it was regarded as punishment from God for immorality and sinfulness. In those days of an imposed religious culture of suppression and repression, it came down to praying, repenting, choosing the established way to heaven or hell - that was it!

And so the local people betook themselves to church to pray more fervently. In the human condition this is a form of cognitive dissonant behavior, namely, the more something has gone wrong or is not working, the more we keep repeating the same behaviors hoping that something will change.

For the Bubonic bacteria, this was its "heavenly" reward. Where people gathered and concentrated, there they thrived and spread. As people prayed more frequently in the churches, the more breathing, wheezing, and proximity contacts, the more the infections spread. So who got out alive? Those who sought to change their beliefs, habits, and behaviors. Those who intuited something else was needed. Get out of town if you could, or get to your country villa, if you were one of the fortunate to have one. Lo and behold, the birth of a new creative minority! Turns out that these are not only the ones who survived, but through that experience, stimulated growing interest and more intelligent behavior. A new awakening away from the life-suffering, punitive mode of a toil-driven, dreary, to be endured not enjoyed, imposition of the divine order to another view of that divine order. Enter appreciation and connection with nature, with the human body, with beauty, knowledge and eventually science. They went on to become change agents, ushering in that once in a many centuries of time cultural explosion that altered the entire face of the society, namely the Renaissance.[3]

Long before contemporary neuroscience was even a blip on the screen, people during the late Middle Ages saw only limited ways out of their life situations of crisis, pain and suffering, and that was: do penance, change your activity, go on a year long pilgrimage, or in the extreme, die for the faith. Sound familiar? Those who went off to do long pilgrimages with many hardships, or to fight in the crusades or other such risky enterprises, were told if they died in such service they would go straight to heaven! Because the plague was interpreted as *poena* - punishment for sinful living, even the many complaints of body pain during this era were interpreted as the curse of Adam and Eve or just living in the "*veil of tears*" planet earth, whose days were numbered.

---

3   Reworked from the author's lectures in European History, University of Massachusetts 1965-67; University of South Florida, 1967-1976

The Pains of Change

We cannot avoid either pain or change in our lives. We react or respond differently according to our level of skill and maturation.

There are at least three ways we can face crises. First, many just react, get worse, collapse, or die. Secondly, some will adapt, learn how to live with it, manage as best they can, and suffer a lot with unpredictable outcomes. Thirdly is the *creative minority*, the ones who respond to crisis, deal with the stresses of life, navigate and transform, coming out better not worse!

There has always been a way to work through crises by eventually transforming negative energies into something more life sustaining. This requires the awakening, organizing and integrating of the body and the mind by listening in to our own organic *somatic* signals.

You can find broad statistics showing what our national physical and mental condition is. In addition to the leading pathologies, cancer and heart diseases, one third of the population is obese, ten percent diabetic, three million have knee, hip and shoulder replacements annually. Osteoarthritis and chronic pain are still on the rise. Even eighty percent of runners develop injuries eventually ending their running.

All of the above involve pain syndromes which in people's emotional lives are inextricably psycho-somatic. Put all the statistics on the major pathologies together and what emerges is that most of the population is living with periodic and repetitive pain. It is also a time of local and global warming changes which for many is painful, especially for the human species.

Repeat pain enough and it becomes a conditioned pattern called suffering. While pain is an unavoidable part of the biological experience, suffering is most often a pattern of adaptation to pain. Shifting out of it is a learned skill involving a body-centered neuro-somatic process of reprogramming.

With the most developed modalities available for treating the varieties of pain from physical to mental (starting with the vast field of medicine, mental health, then physical therapy, chiropractic, acupuncture, massage and so many more, including a host of 'alternative' modalities growing into the hundreds), one would expect the statistics to be showing signs of improvement, with reduction of these painful pathological conditions. That is clearly not the case, indicating a paradoxical situation namely the rise of treatment modalities and new medical interventions coupled with the slowly rising tide of pathologies. Imagine instances when intense rain leads to rivers rising and trying to stop it carrying sandbags. Eventually the river floods. All the above interventions and the health picture show a worsening in our condition.

How long can any society sustain this? Sooner or later disaster will befall us unless we make major changes. Those who do not know how to manage crisis get pulled into reactive fear states which immobilize the body and the brain, conditioning a habitual state of suffering. Those who learn to respond can turn crisis into opportunity and can actually improve the quality of their lives. However, it is usually a creative minority that turns the seemingly impossible or the very difficult into something manageable, easier and more fulfilling. The Renaissance is one major historical example of turning the near catastrophic - the Bubonic Plague - into new unforeseen opportunities. Those who survived had to change their perceptions, habits, behaviors and lifestyle. The Renaissance (rebirth) was a return to principles of nature, a revival of the Greek body-mind-spirit organic connection.

Habit The Hidden Controller
Meets the Angel of Change

Harriet and Harry [species: homo sapiens, the current anthropomorphic self-naming based on our unique ability to know by reflection, connection, inductive and deductive reasoning] are homeowners in the "American Dream" tradition - owning a home with all the sustaining commodities, from food (chickens in the pot) to appliances - a divinely sanctioned prelude, secondary only to paradise's home in the sky!

But heavy rains come, periodically causing leaks, often flooding water into the basement. Harry and Harriet experience significant stress because of the actual damage, and also by the anticipation of further unpredictable episodes. This leaves them feeling helpless against the vicissitudes of nature.

They gradually develop coping strategies to deal with this recurring event, which wreaks damage not only to the basement, but affects the heating, the washing machine and their basement storage. Using basic "sapiens"- given intelligence, they look into water removal strategies and techniques, and soon find someone who is skilled at removing water from basements. Now at least they have found a means to temporarily relieve stress and settle into the habit orientation associated with this arrangement.

But the source remains unresolved carrying with it anxious preoccupation and the continuing irritation of rains producing flood damage. Add to this a host of other concerns of daily life and its dreads connected with this phenomenon. Harry's "sapiens" potential soon gets overloaded, compromised, and suffering begins. He develops high blood pressure, seeks out medical treatment and gets medications to keep it in check. While the decision is seemingly intelligent, nevertheless the medications soon produce side effects which generate more sleeplessness and mental confusion.

Harriet also tries to cope with the situation but soon becomes nervous. Seeking out psychological counseling, she gets a diagnosis of "anxiety disorder," is given anti-anxiety medications, and in this way manages the stress produced by the chain of events stemming from the constant worry around water flooding. Add to this the other preoccupations and toxic anxieties of everyday life - roof leaks, job concerns, relational conflicts, gaining weight - and the stress levels continue to rise. However, they have developed a support structure to help manage mental anxiety arising from these dreaded unpredictables.

Now it happens that concerned friends suggest calling in Sam, an engineer known for his different way of seeing and thinking. Observing the situation

Sam points out that things need not be this way, that there are alternatives that might halt the worsening scenario or even reverse the expected outcome. Sam takes a good look at the entire layout of the land and soon comes up with a plan to resolve the problem. He sees a different path, the key to a prevention strategy, which will divert the water, end the flooding and restore the house to better condition. Harry and Harriet's first response is enthusiastic, open, interested and excited to try this new approach. Sam, however, has to point out that the strategy only works with preparation applied in due course before the actual recurrence of this painful event.

"Oh yes, we will do what it takes. Just show us the way. We're already excited and ready to make the necessary changes. We just need to change our plans and scheduled appointments a bit, then we will be calling you to get started on this new approach which makes so much sense." Sam gets everything ready. Days then weeks go by, but no response is forthcoming. Our habituated homeowners have so many things to do, and so many anxiety-provoking matters to attend to that nothing changes. The old habits continue. What happened?

Harry and Harriet began to realize that this new approach, rational as it seemed, based on good scientific thinking, with a better chance for demonstrable results, would require a change in habits of adaptation. What about the arrangement with the plumber, who was always there to apply the treatment to the flooded basement? And what about this cozy and convenient arrangement with the psychotherapist who offered support and understanding, paid by insurance as well. What would happen if the medications then had to be changed or no longer taken? This better approach, more rational and intelligent as it might seem, involved making a decision to take another path that was unfamiliar and non-habitual. Enter the demon, *cognitive dissonance*. The anxiety surrounding a change in behavior - even though the change augured a more sustainable secure and relaxed way of life - began to mentally supersede the perceived but never experienced benefits.

Habitual Patterns and Changing Conditions

We can talk about change but how to live it and its unpredictable nature is the real challenge. As with any unknown driving force we cannot see the outcome. Some people can't handle it and become conditioned into more pain while others are trying to prevent it. To be living in a time of change is anxiety breeding, often painful. It can also be transformed into creative excitement. One of my well-known professional colleagues confidently expressed to me, *"Crisis? I wouldn't miss it for anything!"*

When you are in the middle of a fast moving river, or worse a typhoon, an earthquake or a civil war, it's another thing altogether. The Greek observer Heraclitus described change as the very way of nature, the rule not the exception. *"You cannot even step in the same river twice!"* The modern forerunner of neuroscience and himself transformed through crisis somatic pioneer, Moshe Feldenkrais, observed that "movement is life." Awareness about how we move through situations is a necessary process bringing our body-mind into sync, improving functional actions at all levels, and providing continuing variations, new sensory-motor perceptions that actually stimulate the brain and improve the quality of life. On the other hand fear of change, trying to keep things as they are, does not work.

The reality is that both constellations of habit and change coexist within us. In the universe of physics, things that do not move or change result in *entropy*. But repetitive habits also exist. Patterns, for example, repeat themselves but never exactly in the same way. No two movements are ever the same. In biology, there is both homeostasis and evolution.

How Pain Cycles Continue

With the development of neuroscience, we now know that any kind of sustained pain is a signal from the brain that something is wrong. A warning to check it out, find out more. Otherwise we might do more damage if we continue in that behavior. Any pain we feel in the various parts of our body comes from the brain and nervous system. If pain signals keep firing, even after applied treatments to reduce them, they must be influenced by something else going on internally. Seeking treatment for temporary relief from pain, most continue to get that relief by returning to the same mode of treatment dispensed in the same location. This is called state-bound conditioning. If the source of the pain is not addressed and there is no change of pattern, treatments become less effective and the pain keeps returning. In my practice I have seen this in many clients. The brain becomes conditioned to be in chronic pain, expecting relief from the next treatment - a closed cycle of vicious repetition.

As observed by Norman Doidge, neuropsychiatrist, *"long after the body has healed, the pain system still goes on firing..."* The once acute pain can become habitual pain. *"Whenever any activity that links neurons is repeated, those neurons fire faster, stronger, and the circuit gets better at pain."*[4] Neuroscience has found that "the brain that fires together wires together." *"The converse is also true,"* Doidge notes, *"Stop doing that behavior and the connections are weakened."* Neuroplasticity, or the brain's ability to change itself, can become either a blessing or a curse. If you learn something and you get pleasant sensations, it's a blessing. If you get painful sensations, it's a curse. In the Middle Ages, where belief, faith and fear were prevalent, the curse side held sway.

So are we really more advanced or at least better off? This depends on your view and your psycho-somatic condition. We no longer see people running around with pustulating bubonic boils, and now we even know better not to congregate and spread it. However, we have created the conditions for pains to persist by *only* treating the pain symptoms. By further fostering a world of conditioned pain

4 From *The Brain's* Way of *Healing*

though kinder and gentler treatments using the now most prevalent use of medications we feed the unsustainable. The expansion to more modes and repetitions of treatment paradoxically perpetuates chronic pain, while simultaneously covering up the pain with even more forthcoming medications and treatments.

The Case of Cora

At age 38, Cora was living seized up with an almost biblical plague of pains and distress throughout the lower back and hips. Once active and movement aggressive (doing the push-pull, try harder mode of exercise and sports activities), she had now hit the wall. Despite many recommended treatments of all kinds, she experienced neither lasting relief nor improvement. From a psychological perspective she was feeling increased anxiety and a sense of impending incapacitation. Medical exams showed, as they commonly do, no identifiable cause but just enough meaningless medical labeling syndromes like incipient arthritis, tendonitis, or degenerative disc disease to fuel more worry and anxiety. She was then sent off with prescriptions for both pain pills and a certain limited amount of conventional physical therapy. [Even insurance companies have found that continuing therapy soon runs into the law of diminishing returns, namely no further improvements through treatment.]

Getting no further help from the medical field, she then turned to the growing consumer culture marketplace of alternative modalities. Hearing about a few who were helped by non-conventional medicine, she visited a chiropractor who diagnosed her with spinal misalignment, the result of "subluxations." She was told this was the cause of her problem — something now disproven by clinical tests and findings! The required treatment was of course an intensive weekly regime to get those mechanistically misbehaving vertebrae back into alignment. And so, Cora opted for and received the recommended treatments beginning three times weekly for at least a year! During treatments she would sometimes experience temporary on-site relief which conditioned her to continually return. The feel-better experience typically but ineffectively happens in the office and lasts only a short time. The patient however comes to identify any relief with a state-bound association to the in office treatment. And as soon as she returned to any of her regular daily life activities the pain resumed. Because she obtained some temporary relief in the initial sessions, she kept going back hoping that yet another adjustment might be the one to miraculously work. When it became apparent that this was not working she desperately looked into other alternatives, tried them, scheduling in multiple yet non-integrated, sometimes conflicting treatment to cover all bases! Whatever relief she obtained lasted only a short time.

By the time she came to me she was depressed, no longer connected into body awareness or any other signals coming through besides the painful ones. The mindset of anxiety had become the driver of treatment. I

---

1   *John Sarno, MD, identified this syndrome as tension myositis. See* Healing Back Pain *and other books by Sarno.*

The Limits of Adaptation

The key question I had to ask was why and how was she not getting better? We are all prone to anxiety and soon imagine the worst for ourselves. Anxiety is a negative expectation. *What if there is something really wrong with me, and no one can find it"* This psychophysical syndrome to first worry, lose oneself in the maze of treatments (which make no internal sense to *cns*), then to go in search of some magic bullet or the desperate cure, is common in people with inexplicable postural pains.

Cora like millions of others had lost the way, lost contact with the internal intuitive signals from within, the path to wellness inherent in her own system and now was dependent upon instruction from outside. She sought out a variety of practitioners who applied with promise that their modality or technique would work, that she must think positive and believe. Rather than reducing anxiety by tuning in to her body she was becoming further out of touch, with diminished awareness, moving away from the perception that she needed. The effect was an actual increase of anxiety. Signals from her central nervous system intelligence that might have been working were now shut off. Her worry mind continued to wander in restless agitation. *Is it my diet? Is it a structural problem? Is it punishment?* Or as some might think, *bad karma,* a sign of something permanent and unfixable?

Had she continued in this vicious cycle of negative-reinforced expectations, the rest of the story might have been a life of living with discomfort, pain, restricted movement, eventually chronic debilitation and yes - accompanying all this psychophysical anxiety - an increasing state of depression. Many have ultimately wound up in that community of chronic back pain sufferers seeking relief at the numerous pain clinics, centers and hospitals and there being taught how to live with pain. That path leads to continuing surgical interventions, increased medications, and ongoing maintenance, a substitute - if one can even afford it - for real functional living. The good news is that she took the other path and now is one of many who have found the way back using a mapped out guided program, a clear and easy way of access to listening to responses and intuitive signals from within. All this is learnable but requires that personal shift.

Where To Go From Here

Cora may be the extreme in the growing drama of more muted sufferers who can live with it and carry on, but always feel the grip of a restricted life. Is this our fate? Is it inevitable, really necessary? Or is there no exit, no escape, as many uninformed realists, and religious doomsday predictors would have it? In this time of incredible technological accomplishments and the proliferation of everything from soup to nuts in the realm of therapy, exercise, health and extended longevity, the question to ask is how or why is there such an increase in the instances of life-compromising and depressing pain and disability. There is no answer from inside the box. The only way is to take the road less seen or traveled when the signals indicate. And the findings of neuroscience point the way.

All these are forms of that second stage of dealing with personal or general crises. Adapting can take on the form of *cognitive dissonance*, a mindset of accepting known sources of suffering as better than risking the unknown and unpredictable ways out of suffering.

It often ends up keeping the pain and suffering going in a suppressed form. Not wanting to see what is (ignorance, or ignoring) can make the arising and passing pains of life become addiction-like suffering syndromes.

We cannot control the stresses of life. Our Bubonic Plague equivalent is slower and more ubiquitous. We can learn the skills of transforming the stresses and pains of life into creative responses, however this cannot be achieved if we are not in control of our own bodies. The only way out is through mindfulness in our physical and functional movements, actions, directions, intentions and decisions in the present moments of everyday life.

Chapter 4
Exercise and the Brain

"Exercise is the single most powerful tool...
to optimize your brain function.
Regular aerobic activity frees up thinking,
calms the body so that it can handle stress much better;
leaves the body stronger and more resilient.
It raises the threshold of the neurons...
and stimulate body-cell repair mechanisms...
more than any other stimuli."[5]

"There is a powerful link between
physical exercise and mental acuity."[6]

We have long known that exercise is somehow good for you. Doctors as well as parents and teachers all recognize this but give mostly only lip service to the practice. Young people tend to naturally do more exercise simply because they are more active - running around, playing, participating in various forms of sports-related activities. But once into the late teens the reality is quite different. First, a far more sedentary life style starts to set in. As we grow older (and in a youth-centered society this means passing age 30) our techno-modern life style becomes one of mostly sitting:

5   Dr.John J. Ratey, neuropsychiatrist, author of **Spark**, The Revolutionary Science of Exercise and The Brain, 2008, p.72 cites the research. See also his book, Go Live!

6   From Scientific American Mind, "Fit Body, Fit Mind", July/Aug 2009The revealing discovery: new research studies show that the brain is maintained, stimulated, and brain cells reactivated through exercise! And that this is its major source!

office work, computer, restaurants, television, movies, events, driving, etc. People start to feel and complain about body pain. Just listen in to conversations, what people discuss in public places often includes episodes of some kind of pain - back, hip, knee, shoulder, arm, or hand.

By age 40, there is a statistically observable pattern, a discernible drift towards decline in physical and mental well-being. In come the medications, the surgeries, and the pain killers (which do not end but only temporarily dull pain while the underlying problem continues). Something is clearly missing in the modern lifestyle: intelligent use of the body and sufficient exercise to sustain all body functions. Just as we are experiencing an ecological crisis, so the counterpart of that crisis begins at home, directly in the body and brain: a crisis in our ability to sustain of our health, wellness, fitness and sustainability. While improving our applied technology, our electronics, our service sectors, are we weakening our internal bio-mechanisms? Our susceptibility to disorders? Our very immune systems?

Brain Food: Learning through Exercise

While most schools in the U.S. have diminished the value of physical education in favor of mental testing, one physical education instructor at the Napier high school in Illinois did something different. He put together an experimental group of willing students to come together and exercise before classes started then wrote it up. The results were astounding. This group outperformed their peers in national math and science exams. The answer was clear and the conclusion that follows: exercise may be the single most potent factor in stimulating the brain, creating new pathways in vital sectors. The experiment has slowly begun to be repeated in several schools across the country but the dominant established habit of severely reducing physical education in favor of sedentary learning still prevails.

The central nervous system is remarkable for tracking, recognizing and communicating. When something is not right, unlike a computer error message, the messages come up in a different way. A continuing experience of pain, strain, aching, stiffness becomes a panoply of stressed body movements, unintegrated, under par, or overworked that will lead to breakdowns, injuries, and to anxious unhappy people who suffer without understanding how and why, without a clue as to what is really happening or how to resolve it. The habit of only seeing from within the confines of the box still prevails. Habituation, dysfunctional repetition of behavior - cognitive dissonance it is!

Once you decide what direction you want to take and you are willing to trust the process, this opens you to connecting through both the body's breathing and movement pathways. Soon you start to have a rudimentary map and a path to follow. While not the territory itself, pathway mapping must be based in physical reality, following the energy path of least resistance and being acceptable at the feeling and mental cognitive level. As if voicing this intention, the brain might be saying just as it does in neural circuitries of all creatures big and small, *I am trying to find the way that will work for you. I am trying to manage the gravitational forces through your body-sensing system so we can feel internally supported, secure, confident, move about safely and freely, do what we need, want and must, ably and effectively.*

While this comes naturally for many creatures, for more developed and evolved beings such as mammals, primates, dolphins, whales, and we humans, better use of self is a continuous learning process. The animal that takes the wrong path may not live to reflect on what, where and how things went off course. We have an unusual propensity to take wrong paths, continue on them compounding dysfunction, then reconsider with awareness and get it right. The key is in the intention: learn how to recognize and then choose the right path, get back on track, be in sync with the flow of current reality. Since the *cns* program potential is already established, it's only a matter of following the paths that work better to reclaim your body. In a very fundamental way you are your body. If you are not in it, who's running the show? Who's minding the store?

Towards a Social Change Paradigm

You are by now already cognizant of the new upcoming social change paradigm without throwing out any of the valuable benefits of the current consumer-driven model. It is a shift from separated to integrated, in some ways new yet what has always been, the integrated approach to good body movement and functional exercise. In the active world of natural living, every creature, most of the time, gets the exercise it needs to maintain itself functionally fit. One exception: we have met the unfit and it is us! How can this be? Why? The answer is complex and can be traced back to our make-up. Because we can mind-create all sorts of imagined and believed activities, we began to live in a *virtual* reality. For example, we can just sit and watch any number of activities happening from television's daily life dramas to cinema, sports and live performances with minimum movement (down to just breathing) and get virtually no exercise. If continued this leads to deteriorating body condition.

But notice how we are also attracted to, fascinated by, and admire those who look good and perform well whether actors, athletes, singers, musicians, dancers or others in any other public-admiring endeavor. We homo sapiens have conflicting paradoxical tendencies: capable of high level performance, accomplishers, yet terribly prone to structural body disorders. There has always been in every society a certain percentage of the population that maintains itself well and fit. Without this we would have fallen into a sinkhole of maladaptation and would not have survived. So it really comes down to intention, choice and practice. We homo saps have the basic components and the capacity for awareness which can enhance exercise and fitness to levels both body maintaining and creatively meaningful.

Out of the Darkness: the Brain Rediscovered

Since 1996 a big change has been slowly entering the conventional and increasingly unstable unpredictable marketplace of health management. A new body of emerging research is showing how the brain - contrary to the medical model and previous belief held by generations of neurologists that the brain cannot renew itself - *can and does actually renew itself.* Neurons that fire together, wire together *[The Hebbian Theory]*. Major changes in the neuronal patterns of myelinizing and in the brain cells are now able to be detected. The implications of a brain that can change itself must also inevitably change the landscape of current expensive and failing treatments.

Biologically Based Exercise vs. Consumer-Driven Varieties

Available studies and statistics show that those who exercise with consistency whether gently or more energetically live longer with less health problems. Lower resting heart rates reveal a correlation with longevity. Larger animals have slower heart rates and live longer, like our elephant, along with whales and others - evolutionary energy efficiency at its best.

We give a lot of lip service to exercising but we do not extend this beyond the socially limited value we have assigned it. After all is said we have more important things to do! But exercise seen from a new perspective and sustained by solid scientific studies is a *biological imperative,* a basic need and activity requiring dedication but also pleasurable, playful, and accomplishing. It maintains all the vital organs, the major and minor body systems. Animals, birds, and many humans engage in exercise as activities of daily life, as necessity, an enhancement, or performance without feeling resistance or being self-conflicted.

When intelligent functioning is lost people will still exercise but view it as an unwelcome intrusion, an additional burden, a task that one must do to alleviate distress, lose weight, stay in shape, and so will grin and bear it. The attitude is more like *I would not be doing this if I did not have to. I don't have time, but if it's necessary, I'll make myself do it.*

Much of the fitness craze often leads not to true fitness but an uncomfortable, achy, even pained body state. Exercise for many has become a necessary intrusion, a time-consuming task, often a distasteful activity, something to do only at prescribed times because it's necessary, otherwise to be avoided. The psychological driver may be a strange form of our mind's disposition to adopt confusing, compensative, often anxiety driven mixed messages. Creating self-motivating and yet self-punishing beliefs such as *no pain, no gain.* The human mind being what it is can easily get recruited into adopting anxiety provoking strategies that seem to provide some temporary adaptation to insecurity - a stress relief cover up! These responses to the stresses of life may increase distress or do damage. Those in the exercise consumer world keep trying out new approaches which seldom lead to a sense of feeling in flow, calm and clear. All these are departures from our inherent psychobiological intelligence which otherwise embraces exercise as natural, sustaining and yes, even enjoyable!

In order to return to the essentials the prerequisites are curiosity, interest and then intention. Can you imagine anyone anywhere - barring fanatics, rigid self-immolating fundamentalists and crazies - who would not be interested or would not choose this path, prospect and potential, were that option made available.

With 80% of the population experiencing some form of continuing episodes of pain, some becoming chronic-repetitive (occasionally acute enough to stop you in your tracks), it's time to look for the way through and beyond. It's available by tapping into the most reliable system of all, what we now know with good science-based research, how the body is designed to function best. The only missing pieces are how to access the system. The instructions are already built in, available in everyone (like the DNA), but has to be activated and practiced to get it wired up properly. [dictum: no neuronal connections, no learning.].

Sometimes we call it instinct or nature. It still comes down to this - we have the means to do what is necessary to live, work and enjoy but it now has to be cast as a presentable learnable program of study, taught early in schools and learned just as easily as children today are able to navigate computers and internet. As with anything desirable, continuous engaged practice is how it happens, becomes real and most importantly, embodied. The brain learns, relearns, and improves through a process known as myelinization, a new learning pattern is established and becomes permanent.

For those interested I call this process *neuro-somatic reprogramming*. The process summarized:

- The activation comes from a nervous system tuned and responsive gravitational forces including all challenges and demands acting upon us.

- The system figures out how to direct forces so that we can get what we need, want, and choose barring the unavoidable such as inescapable injuries, earthquakes, floods, genetic mistakes, disorders, and debilitation.

- The way this all gets worked out is through our brain's capacity to organize experience in patterns and to direct all movement through the most efficient and safe pathways.

Body Movement Mapping: Connecting the Dots

"The capacity of the homo sapiens brain to map almost everything may be the single most important factor in its development, survival, and expansion..."
–M. Merzenich, neuroscientist

When inventor and founder of Apple, Inc. Steve Jobs described how he lived his life and found success, he used the image of "connecting the dots" of his life experiences. What can this mean? It was his way of describing in symbolic and understandable language precisely how the brain works. Connecting the dots refers to how you put things together in order to both see the territory, the path, the development and to act on these. If you want to go from here to there using a roadmap you in effect will find yourself trying to connect one place with another. You will identify one place and then link it to the next in sequence. If you follow the markers or use software (such as Mapquest or GPS systems) you are likely to arrive at your destination. That is also how most brains work.

Getting Ready for the Change Over: Transforming Stress into Health and Wellness

"Life is stress!" -H. Selye, <u>Stress Without Distress</u>

"Health is the ability to deal with stress and come out better."-Moshe Feldenkrais

Our natural and man-made environment is full of stress: sunlight, smog, miscommunications, misunderstandings, confrontations - inescapable conditions which have within them positive transformative potential. From birth on we are responding to the stresses of life adaptation starting with our emotional needs plus the major growth and early developmental challenges like learning how to manage lying, sitting, standing, turning, walking to get from one place to another, getting increasingly better, easier, or faster as needed. All this comes before we engage in sports, exercise and other demanding performance activities! That complex of functions provides enough movement to sustain your life. If you add in more activities such as brisk or power walking, running, jumping, other sports and dancing, you may feel even better, more energetically fit.

In most of our everyday activities we are continuously manipulating things whether it be washing a dish, writing a letter, working on a keyboard or on a computer. What we do, how we organize and move with our hands, arms, shoulders, trunk, spine, hips, legs, feet in all of these functional acts is critical to our well being. Do it wrong and inevitably there will be trouble. Or get it right, however you do it - by trial and error, by curiosity, by intention, by experiment - until it feels complete, connected and satisfying. You are then on the way to a healthy body that now can take you through life with a minimum of pain, trouble, breakdown, injury and all the rest including the variety of the muscular skeletal disorders that seem to afflict mankind.

My observation from clinical experience is that no amount of known externally imposed instructions, medical treatment or makeshift modalities promising the cure to this and that; no TV programs or anything else on how to stay well and fit can match the evolutionary power of the body-brain system. Nor can any of the popular marketed programs on how to stay well and fit - from gym machines to the gym rat's pump-lift-force-stretch-sweat-speed up - match the power of natural functionally integrated exercises. Every child is stimulated by internal developmental movements - instructions from within. Reliance on external instructions would be disastrous. You can assist by modeling but not by a manual to show an infant how to walk.

We are constantly receiving sensory-motor feedback that every creature relies on for all true activities of every day life. But to register this requires tuning into the channels and listening - a big missing piece in school and social education! So begin by getting to know the map of the territory and recognize the common primary core body pathways that all our generated movement energy must take. [See the body mapping system we have developed with specific exercises in our CMI booklet and lesson-exercises available on line.]

We are grounded in a commonly shared world of gravity, bio-mechanics, and physiology. Only by interest or intention can we transform limiting habits and recast them another way. Living in a busy consumer culture without clear directional paths we quickly go off course. By developing both discerning mind and movement skills we can form newer patterns. Just as we use guide maps to travel so we can develop movement maps to direct us. "Know yourself" said Socrates, the Greek philosopher. The modern way of self-knowing is through awareness in the way we move, sense and feel. This time around it will be about learning the body's *gps* to get back on track, to reconnect with the basic elements of our nature, the grounding that underlies health, fitness and well-being. The task is to build a series of bridges that will connect and integrate concepts and practices of body movement, exercise, awareness and intention that have a sound biomechanical and bio-physiological basis and can be shown to be beneficial.

Then it's a matter of walking the talk, taking these ideas into real direct experience. In this way we come to know ourselves in a real substantial way, evaluating and adjusting until we come to trust that what we do is actually good for us and lasting.

Precision Movement Programming

If a primate swings from a tree branch towards a given destination it must have a sense of the trajectory, the force required, the direction and arrival point. Making a mistake means injury, trouble, danger of survival. No doctors around in that realm! It is either recovery or death by starvation or predation.

If a bobcat leaps to try to catch a rabbit, its nervous system is instantly engaged in several internal calculations to determine the approach strategy, the right amount of body/muscle mobilization, the moment of leap and the follow through of speed, acceleration, turns and adjustments. It's trial and error - the way the brain learns. Or with eagle, hawk, albatross, and cormorant tracking a moving fish from a height, they glide, hover, calculate, then dive at great speed, and hopefully strike precisely. The starter rewards are basic need satisfaction. The lesson? Learn well and you thrive!

Now switch the focus to the human species. Get into the body-mind responses, the quantum-like complexity of a tennis player having a ball coming toward you at great speed. In a few milliseconds your nervous system tries to organize to meet and return it. Or you are the server initiating a strategy, hitting the ball at such an angle and placement that your intention is to confuse, discombobulate, and befuddle the opponent. Basketball requires precision moves in order put the ball into a basket under pressure and physically imposing situations. The players must be able to perform a coordinated action, a strategy to execute the play.

In a football game (USA style) the quarterback does not just run or throw the ball. The play has been calculated. Players are assigned downfield positions and specific angles of turning and twisting maneuvers. If all goes as planned the quarterback must first evade the attacking opposition then seek out the tight end receiver, then calculate force and distance, and hopefully get the football into a designated targeted space. Otherwise, the ball is not caught. Worse, the opponents intercept it.

Soccer requires incredible coordination. The individual player may be a high scorer but without the strategic positioning and support, individual prowess would count for little. Soccer along with Cricket attract the greatest amount of spectators (many who have played the sport themselves or just come, sit, stand, leap, cheer - often getting emotionally upset, or angry, if the home team loses!)

There is obviously something psycho-biological and archetypal about these skillful activities which are held in high esteem and involve precision movements and coordination. Something in these activities is so compelling and interesting that spectators (most of whom really need exercise) will pay a lot to see athletes who do not need more exercise. The downside of this social model of staying fit is that these athletes experience both injuries and increased body wear and generally retire early. All we can surmise about the sports attraction and craze is that it appears to be an innate social procliv-ity to be part of a ritual of extreme coordination and collaboration cast in a very competitive style of expression. Whether the primary drive is one or the other is not the main point. Seen from the big picture it's the engagement and the spark that matters.

How It Works: The Physics & Physiological Components Of Good Movement

"Through one path or another all muscles and bones are connected to one another and a change in muscle tension or limb position in one part of the body must be accompanied by a compensating change elsewhere. The system can be visualized as a complex tent-like structure. The bones act as the tent poles and the muscles as the ropes bringing into and balancing the body in the desired posture. The proper functioning of this type of a structure requires that the forces be appropriately distributed over all the bones and muscles."
-Paul Davidovits, **Physics in Biology and Medicine**

Resonance, or motion flow is a process drawn from physics and mechanics, specifically as in resonant frequency of mo-tion: oscillations, pendulum actions, coils and springs, and spirals. We use resonance in the context of organic systems, such as animal and human movement to mean a very specific kind of sequential motion flow involving the reciprocal lengthening and contracting of muscle groups along pathways in which forces are moving smoothly. Whether expressed as oscillating, undulating, rhythmic (like beat in music) or smooth, *resonance* involves a distribution of energy in such a way that every movement we do generates a force and produces energy. The nervous system and body structure seek to direct and organize movement energy into pathways for greatest efficiency and effectiveness by sensing, monitoring, and directing gravitational forces. Generated energy also follows previously learned programs, automatic or habitual patterns, plus new and intentional actions. *Resonance* in brief is the full rhythmic contraction and expansion of the body's muscles and connective tissue (fascia) producing form and shape which the brain records and saves as an image of movement. When we are in resonance we are in a positive state of being which not only feels right but also enhances efficiency in action and performance. It is generally incompatible with pain which is more associated with irregular, turbulent or impacting movement, even with depression or anxiety.

Lengthening is a necessary condition for smooth movement, strengthening, and improved performance. Muscle tissue is designed to maintain residual tone by contracting and lengthening producing force. Muscles acting together produce synergistic resonance. Lengthening extends beyond a single muscle. What is the connective tissue (*fascia)* doing while muscles are lengthening in phase with the contracting muscles? The fascial net links and spreads as the connective tissue surrounding muscle action draws taut, spreads like a sail, shapes like a garment, and gives every movement a definitive form, a structural effect, web of the body including some tough tissue like tendons and cartilage.

All functional movements of the human body lead to a lengthening of the spine in one or more of its planes of movement. Lengthening, as well as contracting, must follow pathways that transmit forces in specific organized sequential waves, the resonance feature described above. Other wise, the body, when not well organized, and when moving with forceful tendencies will tend to shorten. Such shortening takes place in muscle, fascia and joint articulations. Continuous shortening generates many problems. Lengthening is the key factor in release of contracted tissue often related to pain syndromes. It is the basis of good exercise and core strengthening.

Stretching is more local, focused on muscles, and also fascia, best done at the end of the lengthening cycle, and only for a few seconds (but can be done up to 30 sec. maximum, very slowly). Because of the muscle spindle response in the neuromuscular 'wiring,' too much stretching actually sets off a later muscle contraction and is often implicated in muscle-joint soreness and injuries. Some exercise physiologists and sports' trainers claim (always questionable and changing!) that stretching is more effective when the body is warmed up, before or even after an event. Muscles tend to shorten owing to their constantly contracting in the gravity field which then requires more lengthening and some

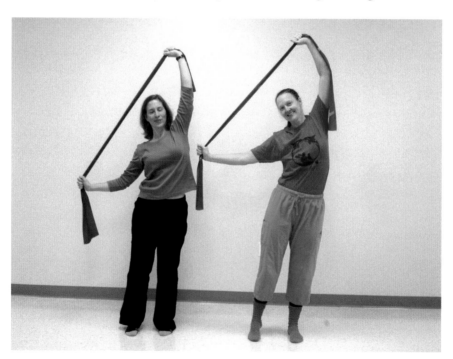

timely stretching. Muscles that stay shortened become too tight. Mobility is now compromised. If done right, stretching stimulates blood circulation and provides temporary relief. In combination with lengthening we can get improved circulation, and some of the elasticity and mobility we need. Animals great and small stretch to a certain extent, usually briefly. Close examination of the movements they do once again reveal that the stretching is really a part of the lengthening sequence. The general guideline then is to lengthen before stretching. Good stretching takes place between muscle attachments, in the middle of the muscle, and not at the tendons. Stretching is done slowly, and is not held long. Stretching is best done at the end point of lengthening, and is helpful in increasing blood flow and range of motion.

Strengthening will take place as long as we are moving in the field of gravity. By increasing the resistance we can promote more muscle fiber growth. Therefore any action against gravity produces some strengthening of muscles. Is it better to do isolated or integrated strengthening? Both have their benefits. Isolated strengthening exercises are helpful in rehabilitation, or for some specific enhancement of performance- as long as you then integrate. It is interesting that animals, which are generally much stronger and fit than most humans, do not do isolated exercises but rather integrated exercises. Strengthening develops as we use the muscles in some playful, purposeful, or intentional action. For example, when the 'great migration' of herd animals takes place in Africa with the dry season, involving long distances to where water can be found, all the animals are prepared. They do not require specific muscle training development apart from what they do in natural daily life activities. This mode of strengthening appears not only more natural and universal, but correlates with a much more functional and structurally integrated body that is able to move better and accomplish more. The distribution of effort allows larger muscles to participate with smaller muscles along specific myofascial chains-pathways that conduct the energy of movement expression.

Core strengthening takes place in key areas following the six primary core pathways. This strengthening is systemic and synergistic: As key muscles along designated paths are strengthened, postural support is also enhanced. Strengthening is therefore combinatorial, sequential, uses levers and balances large muscles with smaller muscles, in tonic and phasic action sequences. All creatures and especially human beings need strengthening but that comes with living and moving in functional ways. In the field of gravity most of our movements are called anti-gravitational, actions that are attempting to keep us upright against forces that are pulling us down. But this is precisely as it has to be, not a battle but a balancing act, a harmonious event. If you find the right movement paths, not only are you able to stay up easier but you get stronger as well.

Relaxation: When the body is in resonant motion flow, so are the breathing rhythms. The effect will be to produce pleasurable sensations, a flow of endorphins , the physiological effect known as the *relaxation response*. The moment of relaxation is essential in all movement activity from daily functions to exercise and performance. Relaxation is not just a mental state but is activated by the resonant quality of movement itself. Movements through the core maximize center of gravity efficiency and require less effort. Relaxation can be felt and practiced in a variety of ways, through slow moving activities from yoga to tai chi, or in fast moving activities including running, walking, and swimming. Through conscious mental activity, through imaging, we can bring about what is called a relaxation response. The key is in the breathing rhythm, the fundamental mechanism that produces a return to homeostasis, or basic balanced state. The more high level athletic activities require finding that moment of relaxation response in order to continue the activity. Relaxation is a function of resonance plus image and intention. When we are in active but relaxed movement flow we can feel a certain contentment, confidence, even commitment, a certain state of body equilibrium, a necessary condition of health and well-being.

To summarize: an intelligent body requires an operating and informational traffic-flow directing system that is sending signals through the muscular chain and to every other part, all in the service of keeping us upright, flexible, balanced and able to respond adequately in the field of gravity. That same body must be able to move up, down, right, left, and sideways, turn and twist, change postural positioning, contract and lengthen, and accomplish what it sets out to do at least enough of the time. The same forces of gravity that can elevate and elongate us also pull us down. When we lose the functional ability to stay up in all daily life activities, the inevitable result is shortening of postural muscles and compressing of joints. This inexorable tendency can be counteracted first by learning to perceptually recognize the state of being upright in standing, and secondly be continuously doing movement actions and occasional exercises in daily life that lengthen the body. In fact all good movements should and do keep the body lengthened and expansive. Animals in nature do not often get tight, restricted, shortened or compressed. To become so would compromise their ability to live.

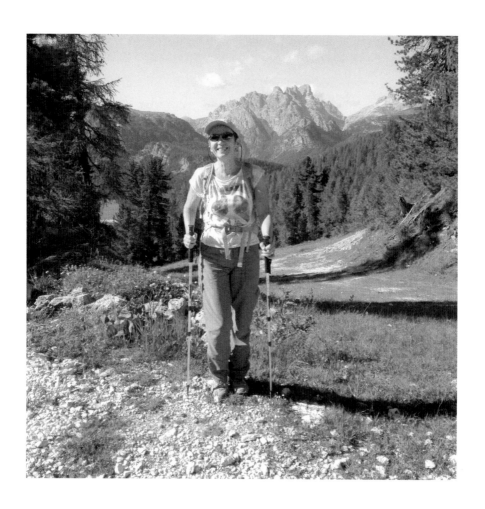

Chapter 5
Born to Walk

The walking experience is primordial. All land based creatures great and small do it. Humans have been relying on this primary functional activity of daily life for as long as we have been around and especially since the Ice Age 70,000 years ago. Without the ability to walk efficiently long and well, homo sapiens might have died out with the rest of the hominids. Some have gone further, developing gait actions into a high-grade level of functional movement and exercise that can combine basic body health and fitness with artistic performance and athletics. Think of running and dancing as an extension of the basic fundamental ability to walk.

The Way of the Walk

What is it in a person's way of walking that looks attractive, draws our attention, resonates with us? It expresses smooth motion flow, has a certain elegance to it, a look of confident directed stride, communicates an image of good body posture, muscle action and coordination, and a relaxed sense of power and ease. Contrast this with walking disorganized in posture, inelegant in gait, perhaps a slight shuffle, grind and slide, signaling disorder, discomfort, difficulty and perhaps a hint of guarding against pain.

"We learn to walk by walking… intrinsically an act in space and time that we generate while becoming ourselves…
It is impossible to be aware of oneself without being able to walk properly, and without knowing which direction to go in…

*Every moment of wonder [stupore] begins by meeting the world,
lifting the feet - moving, dancing, running...*"[7]

- The Philosophy of Walking: Exercises in Mediterranean Meditation, by Duccio Demetrio

*"I will give you intelligence and show you the way which you
then must walk..."* - Psalms 31

It is not so easy to walk as we assume. When robotic engineers tried to get robots to walk, they encountered difficulties so complex that it made calculating its center of mass an enormous undertaking. What took millions of years for humans to develop we take for granted -100,000 sensors just on the soles of our feet! If the hardware and software are not in sync, the robot falls.

Even Elephants Walk Till the Last Day

*He who regrets dying misses the gift of acceptance for having been
born in the first place...*

> *She is now in her 80th year, wandering through the Serengeti with her herd. Tough, stressful and challenging along the way, but on the whole a life fully lived. The elephant is regarded as a very perceptive social animal capable of establishing lifelong relationships even with humans.*
>
> *Our elephant (and all related social animals) senses she cannot keep up with the herd, cannot continue her necessary life activities like foraging, and at some point turns in another direction - towards the ancestral elephant graveyard now a distance away, perhaps many miles. Approaching, she gently touches the remains of those she might have known, grown up with, been related to, and then chooses a spot, lies down, breathes and eventually dies. From all known observations she shows no signs of noticeable distress at all. We cannot know her whole experience but body signs do not lie. And most remarkable, yet commonplace, she walked to the graveyard.*

---

7   **The Philosophy of Walking: Exercises in Mediterranean Meditation**, by Duccio Demetrio, 2005, Milano

Tanzania: We stood silent, motionless as the elephants moved around us. The elephants walked by, seeking good vegetation. I heard about a local man who had some kind of rapport with elephants, and was helping them in their survival endangered by poachers. When he died, the elephants walked around the place where he had lived for three days.

This experience is not specific to such herd animals, even predatory ones. Humans - if they weren't injured, diseased, killed - have been living and *transitioning* this way for as long as we have records. One example I recently came upon at the sight of Canary Islands cave dwellers: when a person felt that inexplicable internal message just like the elephant, they would announce, "I want to die now." They were then brought into a cave, given some milk, and the cave was closed. Even in contemporary rural Switzerland where walking is the primary movement activity, the saying goes, "Walk till your last day!"

Our modern folk, mostly urban and suburban habituated, not only have many difficulties moving with ease, they are mostly unable and unlikely to walk to their final resting place! What has always been a natural biological cycle now gets loaded with additional anxieties about dying. Even the prospects of an afterlife do not seem to calm the inner waters. The myth of a divine order or deity calling for your return still leaves most in some form of restless anxiety. It is our peculiar nature no doubt, the way our brain is configured with its big limbic system making us emotionally labile. From another perspective, being well and fit (*mens sana in corpore sano*) makes the whole process go a lot easier and better.

On planet earth life is stress whatever the driving forces may be. Opportunity or creativity make it exciting, a potential growth experience, rewarding in itself. In western civilization the decline is a difficult, depressing, often one of slow extended degeneration with increasing discomfort, pain, disability and dementias, sustained by more medications, medical interventions, parts replacements and a lot of home or nursing home care that will prove ultimately too costly to continue.

Time to leave the big conundrum and the unknowns behind for the moment, taking with us only the best of the experience and insights of those who have entered some kind of sphere of somatic wholeness and bliss. Living fully embodied, well and fit, has always been not only a state most everyone would welcome (if it just came to you, would you take it?) it also turns out to be a healthy non self-conflicted way to live, an easier less tension-fear driven way to die, that is naturally a transition to the great whatever, "The All There Is" [Stephen Hawking], the god story, cosmic reabsorption, the universe, the oneness sphere, even rebirth!

If priority is given to the skill of moving well, this offers the best outcome. Reliance on anything less is secondary. Treatment, medications, surgeries, and instructions from an outside source are sometimes necessary in an emergency, a lifesaver. Appreciate this huge benefit. Use it to get back on track to the real sustaining bio-logical imperative, the opportunity to "heal thyself" [Hippocrates] which the body does by itself, and better when enhanced with skill-ful means.

Depending primarily on instructions from outside sources is disempowering and highly suspected to reduce much needed brain stimulation as we age, and to generate more plaque. The old ten commandments from a once and still believed divine authority on high, have been now made secular by new commanding authorities who will not even legally allow dying as one might choose, killing is far more acceptable! More later as we discuss the psycho-physical interactions.

Neglecting basic needs, physical and psychological, carries with it serious compromises leading to a long suspected slow slippery slope of "dis-ease" and degeneration. Extending life without quality of life can be a set up for depression, further fuelling degeneration.

As the Greek philosopher Socrates might have put it, "The unexamined life might not be worth the living."

Key Factors: Walk, Track, Love and Trust

We were born to walk. It's primary and universal. Running is secondary and mostly for the young the world over. From Paleolithic to prehistoric to modern, humans have learned to walk well, strong, long, and with endurance.

About seventy thousand years ago all existing human species faced a major crisis, the Ice Age, and with it, scarcity of food. Humans became an endangered species. Biological research strongly suggests that only one group survived and these were our common ancestors. What learned skills did they possess? The hypothesis is sustainable on evidential grounds, and not just speculative.

- First, they must have been able to walk well, efficiently and rapidly carrying light weapons.

- Secondly, they must have developed a special ability to read animal tracks while walking rapidly. Animals at this time were constantly on the move to find food.

- Thirdly, since they could not see what they were tracking, they must have developed a sustaining trust and belief, namely that if they stayed on the path, followed the tracks, engaged in the process without doubt or despair, they would realize the fruits of their endeavors and find their reward, their future.

This suggests the beginning of human psychology, spirituality, and even religion. [See the studies of Peter Underhill, anthropologist and molecular biologist at Stanford University] Our ancestors (related to the Kalahari Bushmen of Africa) learned while walking to read what the animals were doing. The human skill par excellence has always been how to make connections and form a picture.

Animals on four limbs move faster, getting to safety and to where the food is. However, on two legs you are more energy efficient. Our paleolithic ancestors were more tuned, clever and strategic mappers in the making. Homo Sapiens had to be able to both walk, read the markings and track the direction of the animals. In fact, tracking is still done today. But reading tracks is not so easy. It requires focused attention and an ability to follow markings. Sherlock Holmes, the fictional ultimate detective character, is a master tracker seeing what the others don't. "Elementary!" he exclaims to his colleague Dr. Watson.

Without having learned efficient upright walking our ancestral hunters would not have been able to sustain the long stalk-walk needed to find the prey. Reading the tracks correctly means also making decisions as to whether to continue. Tracks reveal an entire world of behavior. Is the animal energetic, weakened, tired, moving slow or fast? While tracking you cannot always see what you are tracking, often for extended periods. Tracking cultivates a sense of trust extending to the love-loyalty bonds of the hunters themselves. It is reinforced by group cooperation, told by night as a tale of the day in a collective act of reinforced group bonding.

Varieties of the Walking Experience: Bushmen to Modern

Walking is uniquely human. The art and action of walking upright with ease, efficiency, and energy to migrate great distances (as during the Ice Age), to go almost anywhere is natural to homo sapiens, yet wondrous and remarkable in its development over time.

Recently there have been several published research studies on walking, including the gait and biomechanics of African tribal women who often carry significant loads on their heads. So efficiently have they learned to walk that the head, neck, and spine stay close to the center of gravity, without bounce, while feet, legs and hips do the propelling. Unique to them - and by extension to Indian and South American women, men not excluded - was their ability to self-organize in such a way that they could maintain erect posture for miles at average speeds far excelling what most people in "advanced" industrial societies can generally do. Despite carrying objects on their head there are rarely 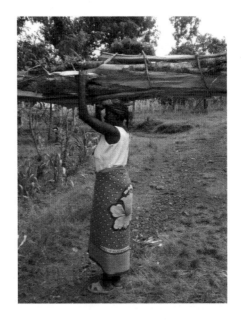 any known cases of cervical strain. A knee, hip or back problem might occur but seldom becomes chronic. What they have learned over millennia is how to sense and organize their walking through what we call sensory-motor consciousness. This comes about by some built-in process involving training *cns* pathways of movement around the center of gravity, the core area where forces are neutralized, the hips, spine and head balanced, the walking gait lighter and smoother.

No pounding, no foot problems, no surgery or radically "corrective" devices needed. From African folk to American Indians, South Americans and Asians, Eskimos, people who had to travel long distances in hot and cold climates and walk at a sustained clip had to learn ease, efficiency and resistance-free gliding movements. We now know this had to do with learning to arrange their movements so that their legs, and especially the hips with the larger rotator muscles could perform powerful energy generating actions. Hip joints, pelvis and pelvic floor have to be in connected alignment, synchronized into directional pathway actions with the spine, ribs, and upper body shoulder complex. Generated (kinetic) energy can then be transmitted up through the spine following a spiralic pattern. Verbalized descriptive images are of course just fingers pointing compared to the real internal somatic feel of a good walking experience. Though the images of any graceful, natural, or supportive activity can be appreciated and enjoyed in the viewing, there is nothing like knowing it from the inside, having a "feel" for it. You must experience the quality of flow, the resonance, the rhythm of motion. The talk must be walked, felt, and embodied in ourselves.

Benefits of Walking

"The basic foundation of fitness… studies show improvement in metabolic functions, reduced risk of heart disease and stroke, regulation of high blood pressure, reduction of arthritis; heightened immune resistance to common colds, plus a host of other benefits to the entire body. Walking improves the efficiency of the heart and lungs, burns fat and calories, builds muscle and bone strength. Unlike running, dancing, and related activities, walking is easier on the joints and the back, and walking strengthens more muscles than running… and is a safe exercise for joints that may have been damaged. There are no injuries [let it be noted] named after walking, and it has the lowest dropout rate of any exercise."

- Gary Yanker, exercise specialist,
cited as a founding father of walking exercise.

Walking Requires Skill

Everyone has an imagined, seldom accurate, explanation of what is wrong, from "it's my back, or, my foot, my ankle, knee, hip," to "it's arthritis," "my age," "my genes." Most of the time the problem is not about structural damage, some innate deficiency, or genetic dispositions, but about stresses coming from dysfunctional use. As a movement-centered therapist who has long enjoyed the varieties of the walking experience - hiking, trekking, race walking, and even running - I have, as with many others, experienced pains with no medically identifiable *structural* cause. Since discovering, relearning and practicing a more integrated and efficient walking form, most of the problems have self-resolved. With this reprieve and reversal, like the proverbial cat with nine lives, I have entered a new period of being able to both enjoy and benefit from this health-enhancing, nutrient rich exercise. This personal re-training enabled me to then work much more efficiently and effectively with clients who were experiencing pain and difficulties relating to walking, changing their frame to see from outside the conventional closed box - a different strategy to resolve problems and improve clients' movement patterns.

Making the Improbable a Reality, the Difficult Easy, or How One Person Improved Dramatically in Just Six Weeks...

Testimonial: *"After coming in last (in a Summer series weekly walkers 3.6 mile event), I changed my approach, took Josef Della-Grotte's suggestion and began training with two objectives: improve my form and my aerobic conditioning.*

Between races I trained, steadily increasing my distances until it equaled the distance of the race each Thursday. I remained focused on form with faith that speed would follow incorporating three technical tips JD always tells his racers: stay over your center of gravity; roll smoothly through your feet, spreading and relaxing; rotate from your core levers getting uplift into your spine. I walked, sometimes ran (for the first time in ten or more years), bicycled, cross-trained at every opportunity and took good care of my body.

Finally, on race day I drafted behind a group of three women in front of me and mimed their pace like a mantra, a meditation in motion supported by gravity. For an hour, the duality between the asphalt of the road and the spinning of my feet morphed into a trampoline-like spring rejoicing beneath each foot. I finished close behind the leaders - 20 minutes faster in time than just six weeks ago..."

- Fred Goodwin (writer and poet)

From My Personal Journey (Part 2)

We can talk about walking intellectually and abstractly citing all the research "till the cows come home." What I want to also include here is a piece from the real experience of walking the Himalayas, the Ngorogoro Crater in Tanzania (Africa) and later the Camino Santiago in Spain and France.

The **Himalayas** posed a real challenge. Get in trouble and the only way down was several days by yak. I was also slowed down to a near halt by the increase in elevations from Lukla [9383 feet] on up to Thangboche [12,700 feet] and then to Kala Patthar, the pilgrimage ascent [18,000 feet], described in the following way: *"The walking has a positive effect on the body and the soul, and therefore the trek also is a kind of therapy to bring both the body and mind again in a healthy balance."*

This opened me to awareness in taking each step in the most efficient way. Gravity and physiology speak loud and clear, gait and breathing coordinated. I became extremely proficient and eventually could walk distances with no distress. At the same time the sheer magnitude of isolation (walking alone much of the time) requires being present, moment by moment. Weather changes alone could be critical. No wonder people in this region developed high levels of awareness through walking!

The Himalayan trekking experience, much shorter than the Camino, was simply far more intense. At those altitudes, no stores, no options, and a diet of gruel, rice, some beans, very few vegetables, yak milk and tea. What I learned was the skill of walking and self-management and more.

Walking with a Maasai guide in **Tanzania (Africa)** was less of a great challenge than it was a close-up, hands-on feedback to the way they walk. Even their independence is conditioned by their ability to walk well. They are known as the "ships" of the Serengeti as they glide by at a continuous pace of about 3.5 mph. Because of a one-to-one connection, I was able to map out how they walked, what part of the foot they landed 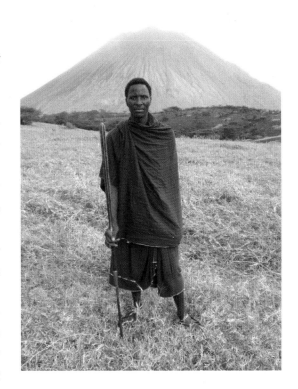 on, the glide-through actions of hip to upper body. My guide John was in his twenties, had ran up Mt. Meru, and could, he claimed, walk a marathon distance (26 miles) everyday if necessary. [To raise funds for his tribe he was willing to come to the States and do just that but getting him a visa was a near insurmountable obstacle.]

At day's end in a village campsite I invited him to do a fast walk of 3km with me, the big age difference of 50 years notwithstanding. While at 5-6 mph I was breathing fast and sweating profusely, he simply adapted his walk, hardly straining in the least, staying near and watching me somewhat curiously. I was reminded of seeing domestic dogs enjoying a brisk walk while the human companion was puffing away close to maximum cardio level.

In the **Kilimanjaro** region, I walked with Chaga tribesmen mostly all up or down. They carry large bundles of grasses from the fields on their heads for their animals while walking at a slightly slower but similar pace as the Maasai herdsmen. Carrying nothing more than a small pack, I could not keep up with any of them,

Another myth exposed: do these tribal people unlike us die much younger? Not at all. From infectious diseases, yes, but those that survive can live well into their 80's. The mother of my guide could out walk me at any time, and had no knee or hip problems. In terms of body sensing and postural alignment, they are finely tuned!

The **Camino Santiago** in Spain and France presented less of a survival challenge. You can stop at any time with a relatively easy means of getting back to some travel access point. It was more of a long extended distance adaptation, factoring in my age as well. Body condition, alignment, uplifting vectors of force, gait and stride became the major considerations if one is to complete the determined number of kilometers planned to arrive at the next destination. My first stage of the trek was 22km daily on average (half a marathon distance). Because of the problems previously described, especially the backpack weight, this goal was effectively reduced to about 20km. Efficiencies and deficiencies at every level would be telling.

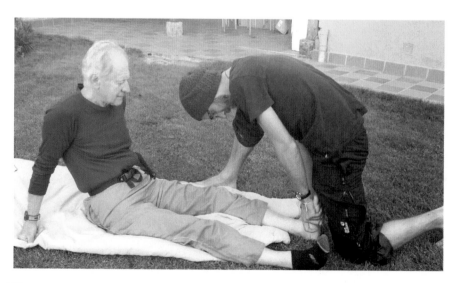

Several times during the day I would have to stop, stretch, slowly do movements and other internal alignments to keep going. I recall at one point barely making it to a town, hobbling over a small bridge when another pilgrim (*pelegrino*) with full backpack asked if I needed help. Turns out he was a Polish born physiotherapist working in Germany! Right there on the bridge he began working on my knee, lower leg, and ankle doing myofascial release maneuvers [see photo] enough to get myself to a hostel *(albergue),* rest, and continue the next morning. This happened a few more times as we met along the way forming a personal connection.

At another time I stopped, took shoes off, and began self-treatment applications, still 3km from the next town. A Spanish pilgrim passing by offered to carry my pack along with his to the town! I demurred but was so inspired by the offer, the very ethos, the *agape* spirit of helping one another (a tradition since the Middle Ages) that I was then able to continue arriving late in the day but okay. Next day the same routine - and yes, I could have taken a day off, but never did. One of the reasons is that staying at any *albergue* one has to be out either early, or if in a private one a little later. This way everyone has to keep moving! Going slower I could now almost keep up, stay in contact with my traveling caravan of pilgrims, and arrive in the same distant village later. One good thing was no forced competitive hurrying (some do the Camino as an athletic challenge, up to 40km daily!) Taking a day off also meant eventually mixing with a new group at the albergues. I was already forming attachments, even though for most of the day I walked alone, meeting one or more along the way and stopping for lunch or a needed rest from the pace.

A further observation: so many of these were having problems of blisters, knee, and hip joints, never having been properly prepared or schooled in the skills of walking. Western urban and suburban people just walk. There is rarely any formal training. And yet it is clear that walking is a skill that needs developing, precisely because we no longer walk the way our ancestors did, nor even close to tribes people like the Maasai. I estimate 25% of those who start on the Camino unprepared will have problems from minor to major. I worked with at least 15 I met just casually during that first one month of trekking.

Some Backup Research Projects

A few years ago at a biomechanics lab, and then later in conjunction with a thesis project (at Worcester Polytech Institute, Mass.) we conducted a series of research studies using biomechanical testing instruments. The results of this study helped us improve our somatic technology, allowing for more predictable positive outcomes with clients in a shorter time. Our practitioners and students could move beyond just applying remedial treatment. It is seldom that only one isolated part - whether the foot, the knee, leg, hip, or lower back - is the cause of the problem. Treatments that only address structural release or limited area rehabilitation relief, statistically show little by way of improvement in the walking gait. After a while, the hidden became obvious, and the observation was once again reconfirmed - namely, that all components of movement are designed to act as one integrated functional, structural and psychophysical entirety.

The Actual Biomechanics of Walking

"Talent is not born in us; it is grown."
- Daniel Coyle, **The Talent Code**

From the time each child gets to standing and begins to walk the *cns* is active, awake, and listening in, myelinizing the child's trial and error experimental inputs that will eventually lead to relatively good balance, support and forward motion flow. A pattern is in process of being formed, then hard-wired for a lifetime of application.

Previously believed by the most eminent researchers to be unchangeable once formed, we now know the programs are modifiable. The impulse for improvement is also built into the brain. In short, new learning is possible. As the child finds balance it also finds pleasant sensations and rewards, able to go here, there, to new places. How all this happens is a complex process learned by doing, but the mechanism is still only partially understood. However, we can develop a map and pathway markers to guide us.

Like any directional map the reading is the easiest part. The map tells you how, where, and what. It's the implementation, the actual doing that counts. There is no other way. The mapping function of the *cns* goes on whether we know it or not. But if you know how to use the map you will get far more mileage and benefits, it will keep you tuned and on top of the game, that is, on top of the life-vitality chart.

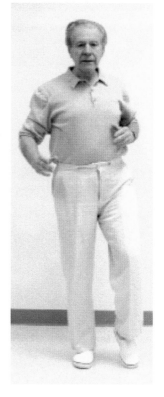

So here is what we rediscovered among the ruins and the ruined: walking by initiating with the most effective movement sequencing works the best. [We named this the path 3-4 sequence. See booklet and DVD promo on walking, also on our YouTube site.] We can learn what comes naturally to most lifetime walkers all over the world, to follow the sequencing signals as all animals must be doing while maintaining dynamic core stability and using spiralic motions. The mechanics are clear, even if lost in life style, that this pattern of initiation is the most evolved, functional and motion-powering pattern of action for a biped who needed, from prehistoric times, to stand erect and move with energy efficiency.

There are six vector movement pathways we discovered and mapped out. Learning them all provides gear-shift options while walking on varied terrain. Central to good walking is what we refer to as Path 3, the basic core stabilizing and vertical spiralic alignment path. Once learned you can use them all in combinations as needed. This can also be upgraded into what is known as race walking, an Olympic sport that was developed by the English (most likely from observing tribes people all over their occupying Empire).

An interesting function related to standing: tribes people the world over and from time immemorial have been observed to stand longer on one leg rather than two. On two legs we are unstable and need to move. On one leg you can align much easier along the gravity line and stay there longer. You might have seen pictures of the Maasai herdsmen or Australian aborigines who can stand on one leg, hold a spear, and remain longer than you or I can wait to check them out! Try it out for yourself.

From Natural and Developmental to Learning and Training

Walking takes place in human beings through developmental stages growing into full maturation unless inhibited or fixated. How one walks will be determined by body structure and imprinting by imitation of peers and elders. Early walking is homologous, a simple balancing act, meaning basic shifting of weight to one side then the other using a form of lateral action like a pendulum. This soon develops into the more efficient rotational, homolateral, or transverse pattern that allows for both counterbalancing and increase of velocity. Notice how young children quickly move around, often faster than adults can get to them. From the pathway mapping system perspective what we see in a child who has entered the developmental rotational stage of walking is a definable path. Looking at a fast moving active child what we are likely to see through a slow motion camera is the pattern we have rediscovered and identified.

People who walk well organized and fit appear to be on the edge of gliding over the surface with a light rebounding touch of the feet. Such people can be seen in certain sports and performance fields moving gracefully and efficiently, staying upright, body spread out expansively. The good news is that walking well and fit is relative, available to almost anyone young or old, requires no specific speed nor distance, and is an activity you can do and enjoy for a lifetime. Cultural inhibitions about moving the hips, especially for women, may produce psychophysical disturbances interrupting the natural tendency of resonant motion flow.

Walkers who learn how to access this pathway of vector energy experience as we pointed out, an uplifting sense of motion flow with elongation of the spine and the neck. It may be less about nature, less in the genes, and more in the nurture that reveals the secret of how certain people look tall and beautifully extended in just walking, dancing or cultivated performance activities. While the very design of our body makes this possible, the program stil has to be activated by both doing and ongoing learning. Then and only then can we human beings walk naturally upright and true.

Research Results: Want to Live Longer, Walk Faster Some Say...

One research study at the University of Pittsburgh claims that your walking speed can tell a lot about you - including your life expectancy. Nine studies that ran from 1986 to 2000 investigated the relationship between walking speed and life expectancy in senior citizens.

The results revealed a clear link between the two variables, the researchers explain (synopsis):

"Amazingly, your walking speed is just as good an indicator of how long you'll live as your health history, smoking habits, and blood pressure combined. It's possible to do a basic life expectancy calculation

based on a person's age and gender, but there's no real way to know how accurate that estimate is for any given person without knowing more about his or her medical history. You can figure out a more detailed estimate by combining information about a person's chronic conditions, medical conditions, blood pressure, body mass index, and hospitalization history, but it turns out you can get just as good an answer with ten feet of pavement and a stopwatch.

Predicted years of remaining life for each sex and age increased as gait speed increased, with a gait speed of about 0.8 meters [2.6 feet]/ second at the median [midpoint] life expectancy at most ages for both sexes. Gait speeds of 1.0 meter [3.3 feet]/second or higher consistently demonstrated survival that was longer than expected by age and sex alone. In this older adult population the relationship of gait speed with remaining years of life was consistent across age groups, but the absolute number of expected remaining years of life was larger at younger ages."

Simply looking at a person's age, gender, and walking speed is as reliable a predictor of life expectancy as any other known method. Admittedly, estimating life expectancy is still an inexact science, but it's pretty awesome - and maybe a little disturbing - that there's such a simple way to estimate how many years you've got left. But why is walking speed such a powerful indicator? The researchers have an idea:

"Walking requires energy, movement control, and support and places demands on multiple organ systems, including the heart, lungs, circulatory, nervous, and musculoskeletal systems. Slowing gait may reflect both damaged systems and a high energy cost of walking."

Now, a person's health is obviously a complex thing, and it's not as though a person's walking speed can magically reveal everything about a person's constitution. That said, it probably wouldn't hurt to try quickening the pace every once in a while.

Some Further Commentaries for Those Interested in How to Walk Fast and Efficiently

There is a growing trend in western industrial and technology based countries, expressed mostly in the fitness and sports sector, towards a kind of power walking. It is often seen performed in a body-forcing manner, but without the elegance and efficiency of the African gait and stride. This trend may have been inspired and sparked by traditions of old such as those Viking-like power-walking styles from Sweden, Finland, Switzerland and other countries. Another form, race walking, is more of a niche sport requiring more training and with stricter rules of leg straightening, especially in competition. However, this and other related forms (which do allow for the natural knee bend tendency) show significant reduction in knee injuries.

Both race walking and varieties of fast walking can often resemble jogging, the difference being that in true walking form one foot always is on the ground, while in jogging both feet are for a moment off the ground. The incidence of structural injuries in walking is far less than in jogging or running because of the significant reduction in both knee rotation and landing impact.

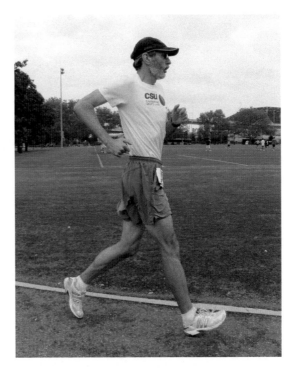

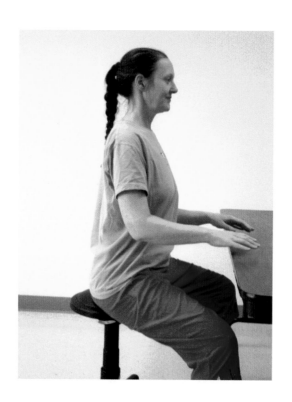

Chapter 6
The Sedentary Sitting Epidemic

"The sedentary character of our modern life style is a disruption of our nature… posing the biggest threat to our survival." - John Ratey

Sitting: Staying Upright, Easy and Supported, or Sagging?

We have been a long time into the era of the sedentary way of life which not so long ago was regarded as desirable progress in living a more leisurely life style. Now it's being revealed to be a slow body degenerating downslide with more lying in soft chairs, furniture and more sitting just as a way of life - all reducing much needed movement stimulation. Continuing research studies and findings show a correlation with a number of disorders and diseases, a setup for deterioration of body and brain.

Let's first review how we got into the mess in the first place. The observation can and has been made that our way of sitting is the primary problematic postural misuse of ourselves in modern times. We sit to call, text, e-mail, surf the web; for recreation (television, movies, video games, plays, concerts); for shopping (via the web); for transportation (cars, buses, planes, trains); for spiritual needs (meditation, attending church); for deskwork and to fulfill other basic human needs. We often spend the majority of our waking hours sitting. During those many hours how many

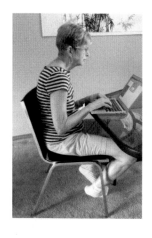

of us pay attention to how we are sitting? Usually we notice what we are doing only when it becomes uncomfortable or painful. Resting on our tailbone it's easy to slouch the spine. Attempting to "sit up straight" (long in use as a verbal prompt by parents, relatives, teachers but very slim on results), most people fall into the default habit of contracting the back muscles. This does not last to stay upright as the muscles fatigue and slouch returns. Or some learn to keep the back tight, which will result in eventual back pain. We may use various pillows and props to maintain a natural alignment of the spine (if it is still available). Almost invariably we rest our backs against a surface.

Poor sitting habits get wired in. The real core pathways of alignment and support for maintaining upright comfortable sitting posture are now compromised, contributing to the widespread weakness of the core muscles, as well as the difficulty in accessing them. Add in to all this overstressed and shortened back muscles.

"Poor sitting habits - especially in the workplace - may be the single most significant factor in back pain, shoulder and neck problems, and even carpal tunnel."
- Sitting is a Killer,
British Research Report

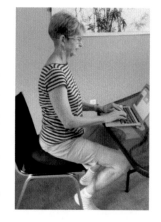

People, like dogs and cats and other creatures, sit for long periods of time. But unlike these other creatures, our sitting mode may be more like pelvic immobilization and spinal sag, more like a sedentary state accompanied by a significant reduction in the minimum daily requirement of exercise to stimulate our natural upright reflexes. Recognition that the sedentary mode was causing problems led to the emphasis on getting more exercise by going to gyms, running, etc.

The Downside - and Downslides - of Sedentary Sitting

Sitting for long periods of time is likely to be a lifestyle habit lasting well into the foreseeable future. Many animals can sit for certain periods of time. But there ends the difference. On all fours sitting is more supported and relaxing, more of a spreading out into a lying position. These creatures also get a lot more exercise naturally, not reluctantly. Our chair style of sitting is more like a plant yourself down state of immobilization. In sedentary sitting most of the body's energy pathways and flow become sluggish, and deactivated. It has now apparent that sedentary sitting is connected with low back problems. But the recommendation to just get to a gym and work out, run or even swim, does not change the configuration that gave rise to the problem in the first place. Soft and backward tilting seats, and those that have what feels like a sinkhole - especially in cars and sofas - prevent movement flow.

Sinking the pelvis stops its motion. Energy forces are restricted from going up. What also happens is that all the other stabilizing muscles of the spine and parts of the brain slowly begin to go inactive. The first automatic response of the body to this weakening is to pull oneself up, engaging the most available superficial back muscle complex. But by working less efficiently and harder they also get shorter. Being shorter they are weaker, and therefore must work harder, which eventually leads to back pain, stenosis, or spinal immobility even without the pain. And then another consequence: a shortening of the entire back muscle chain from the calves to the hamstrings. Most people who sit too much this way can no longer bend forward and touch the floor without forced stretching which either causes pain or muscle cramping.

Before long this shortening compromises and affects one's entire postural equilibrium making not only sitting but then standing up even more difficult.

[Learn how to turn it around with the *Dynamic Sitting Exercises* DVD by Josef DellaGrotte or the new CMI booklet-manual of exercises *Core Movement Integration: Introducing Six Pathways to Lifelong Fitness and Wellness* by Kimi Hasegawa, PT, certified Core Integration practitioner. Both are available at our website http://www.dellagrotte-somatic.com]

Core Centered Sitting: Stable and Supported

"Sitting is a potential athletic activity." -Lionel Wolpin, MD.
"Sitting: It's More than You Think"

We know that sedentary sitting can be turned around, even transformed into a beneficial exercise. Consider that most of the human functional sitting experience over time has been to sit in some kind of moving fashion: squatting, sitting on a rock, a tree, a bench, a horse, a cart, with the basic support provided by balanced motions of the pelvis and spine. That means sitting has been an active daily experience even when apparently nothing much seems to be happening.

It appears at first difficult, almost formidable, to not only change the dysfunctional habits but also all the apparatus, the furniture, the desks! But just as with walking, there are several suggested ways to better sitting including everything from ergonomically designed

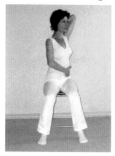 seating, to doing yoga posture practices first, and now to doing much more tailored core-supported dynamic movement exercises while sitting. This involves a shift to a different image and feel, away from the familiar ingrained habit - an upgrade that adds far more value and can vastly improve the actions of sitting upright,

more towards the way we are designed to be. This approach will improve both the body and the quality as parts of the total sitting experience once we know what functional sitting is all about. To improve sitting means to have an available, connected and felt self image of the act and actions while sitting. The base of support to sensing uplift without any forced actions comes from small internal movements to larger more global ones, all becoming integrated into one's self image.

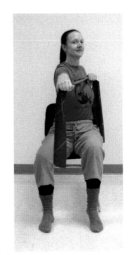

You can start by doing any number of common exercises involving uplift, rotation of the spine, side bending, spreading the arms, bending forward. Apply what you have learned and use it in sitting. Look for classes or programs that emphasize such exercises, the kind that make you feel more upright, supported and strong. Sitting exercises follow the same principles of muscle physiology and biomechanics as any other kind. As long as you are core-organized, moving and feeling ease in alignment and uplift you are getting stronger. The sequence of movements in line with the body and its levering actions activates lengthening and contracting. When there is enough lengthening through the spine and ribs one just stays up naturally. No need to force, tighten or struggle. Muscles are naturally being strengthened along the body's pathways.

Sound difficult? Any of those tribal folk I met along the way would get this fairly quickly, more by just showing, not by the words! And, what if we started to teach this in elementary school, by demonstration and example? By sitting and moving differently, the habitual dysfunction and the postural stresses can be changed, the old problems associated with it eliminated.

Lessons from the East: What the Buddha Knew About Sitting That We May Not

"There is one thing that, when cultivated and regularly practiced, leads to deep spiritual intention, to peace, to mindfulness and clear comprehension, to vision and knowledge, to a happy life here and now, and to the culmination of wisdom and awakening. And what is that one thing? It is mindfulness centered in the body."
- Gautama Buddha

This is close to all we got from Gautama about the actual body involvement in the practice of sitting. From several research studies and my experience working with problems in sitting postures over several decades, I feel closer to knowing more about how he must have developed and sustained his own sitting posture. As with any effective learning through the body as a dynamic system it takes practice and staying on course. Sitting posture is the vehicle that carries everything else. The *body* is from the view of neuroscience a "dynamic processing system." Once we split mind from body we find ourselves in just another state of dissociation and confusion (what the Buddhists and Hindus would call a *dharmic* predicament with some suffering: *samsara!*)

What was the physical foundation of sitting practice in these meditation-oriented Eastern traditions? From my working experience as a therapist and movement educator I view sitting practice as a core-supported process of integrative movements. Whether we are aware of them or not, balancing and supporting muscles are firing continuously. Otherwise we would just collapse. Sitting practice was and continues to be the way to get separated body-mind parts back together and experience a state of integration, deep relaxation, and centeredness.

Observe the classic consistently standardized image of Gautama the Buddha in sitting posture. as represented in statues and stone carvings. He appears comfortable erect, relaxed, no signs of strain, and conveys a state of body-centered mindfulness. How did he get there? First and foremost, he was part of a more body conscious culture, a trained athlete, warrior and a strong walker. His central physical practice and that of these early Buddhists was walking relatively brisk and steady for long distances.

Upon examination right sitting is dynamic. Even breathing contributes to this action. The result is then expressed in language such as effortless, upright, or moving with ease, which in the language of modern physiology would be called efficient postural equilibrium. Otherwise there would be continuous disturbance with eventual degeneration and stiffness in the pelvic region and lower back. This is what seems to happen with many who just sit without the skill set (evident in many meditation centers as meditators practicing *awareness* do continuous sitting often without proper instruction or prior preparation, ignoring the actual postural configuration and state of their bodies.)

Back pain is no stranger to those who sit holding themselves upright by unknowingly overworking the back-spine muscles. Even meditation divorced from its roots in movement and exercise, with too much sitting does not escape the body's reactions. (Such long sitting practice and reduced exercising and concomitant reduced exercise has also been correlated with cancer, "the meditators disease" as it is often called in the East.)

Even our preoccupation with the mind in all it's described forms, but divorced from the body system that informs, it is not only absurd but biologically incongruent. They go together forming the neurophysiological basis of awareness itself as a state of perceived sensations, contrasts and connected knowing, enabling us to witness our physical, mental, and emotional patterns of behavior. It is interesting and synchronistic that neuroscience, physiology and biomechanics have finally struck a chord with a new generation of Buddhist teachers including the Dalai Lama. The brain and body are so involved with mental processes that separation is no longer an arguable option.

Observing and Working with Active Sitting

Dr. Lionel Wolpin describes how he would *"observe patients in the seated position of relative rest and while also moving in all directions… taking a history and examining… to determine the cause and treatment of neck, shoulder girdle, low back and lower extremity pain."*

My colleague, Renzo Ridi, M.D. in Florence, Italy does a full biomechanical testing on equipment plus an elaborate comprehensive intake assessment with his clients. Structure reveals patterns. [Practitioners of Core Movement Integration do a full assessment of clients and students in their seated postures.]

Consider that sitting has many functions. By emphasizing different elements active sitting can be adapted to any situation from meditation and relaxation to play or the workplace. Active sitting can sometimes appear contained and still, or expansive and dynamic.

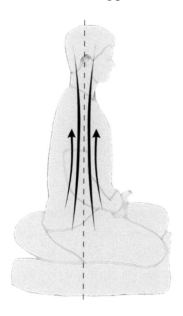

The most important thing is to sense and read the pattern of movement, observe breathing rhythms which track with the primary core pathways, link into the psychosomatic expressions or manifestations, and help open more gateways to relaxation and response. In conclusion, active integrated sitting is an internal experience derived from mindfulness of the body, awareness of sensations, and from the intention to focus and engage. Going into passive slump mode is no longer a viable option!

Chapter 7
Psycho-Somatic Connections:
Where Body & Mind Meet
Emotions, Feelings, Concepts, Beliefs

"Emotions move like a river of molecules targeting specific locations"
–Candace Pert

The interconnections among feeling, thought, belief, body posture and good (or bad) functional movement has long been intuited, much written about but rarely demonstrated on a scientific basis. Yet it has been actually known for some time that there are "final common pathways" in the body system. [As defined in *The Medical Dictionary* 1- the motor neurons by which nerve impulses from many central sources pass to a muscle or gland in the periphery; 2-any mechanism by which several independent effects exert a common influence]

What does this mean? According to this long time standing neurological hypothesis, the wiring is such that any feeling or belief must travel along neuromuscular pathways that express that quality. In other words, feelings are not abstract and disembodied. They are not only in the body but are also expressions of the body in gesture, posture, attitude, behavior and patterns of action. The basis of the *final common pathway* findings and hypothesis is simply this: *any behavioral pattern, whether it is emotional, conceptual, or physical, follows certain pathways that manifest it, internally or externally.*

[See Candace B. Pert, *Molecules of Emotion: The Science Behind Body-*

Mind Medicine, 2000. A host of bio-scientists and neurologists, from Sherrington to contemporaries such as Antonio Damasio, Alain Berthoz, Norman Doidge, John Ratey, and others recognized the direct body-mind connections, interactions, and effects.]

Our concepts about anything and everything follow body pathways. If you have learned and programmed yourself to see the world a certain way, you have then formed a psychophysical path. That is how it manifests. Your body actions, your movements, your gestures and your posture will express and reflect this. People who know how to decode will be able to see and understand where you are coming from. What you say in words is just code language for what you believe and how you see — yet another reason and caveat to never rely on word descriptions as reality! People can use the same words, a shared language to express totally differing perceptions and concepts. All language has to be *decoded*, that is, interpreted by looking at body expression sometimes subtle gestures or shaped expressions which are revealing what the person really means. And often the person may not be necessarily aware at all.

Working with Feeling States

Whenever there is a continuous persistent bad feeling syndrome about almost anything circulating and repeating in the mind's neuro-circuitry it is slowly firing it's way to becoming a wired-in preoccupation, easily morphing into a fixation. Feeling states can be triggered by a variety of stimuli - personal, relational, social, political, economic, or just about anything else that generates restless concern. The big ones are the suppressions, self-conflicts, ambivalences, and agitations that are not channeled, energized and re-directed into some form of positive action or wholesome resolution. These are different from natural emotional recoils and responses from clear and present danger, or from challenging situations that require taking action. When reactivity is being generated by a *negative emotional ego state* (a programmed personal story version that may not correspond to reality) that soon gets rooted internally and subconsciously. The emotional drivers behind the scene may remain hidden but the body never lies. It is revealing by its postural markings. Living with negative emotions (defined as conflicting intrusive energies) produces body reactions which can manifest in a host of disorders. When our energy states turn negative we are driven into discomfort, pain, and ultimately into one or more of the many forms of illness. These negative emotional self-image drivers are resentment, anger, fear, anxiety and guilt.

The point is how to cultivate **somatic empathy,** meaning that you can enter into a person's world, listen, join in, walk with them a while, but not buy into it. Not just avoid, bypass or gloss over things. Empathy allows for openings, opportunities to bring out the dark and the suppressed which when recognized and worked with has value. Obstacles to seeing what is, how things are may also be holding the energy, the key to where the action is, telling the story, and pointing the way through to the fulfillment of the unmet need, taking the skeletons out of the dark, the shadows, the closeted. You can always tell after a while of observing whether a person is in stuck mode, with no viable alternatives or choices. In this way you are aware of the paths of feeling, interpreting and perceiving that the person is in, which is an enormous advantage. On the other side, when we are in a state of clear intention, we feel at ease, confident, open, and available for contact and connection. The nervous system would prefer *intention* because it's about being in the here and now, and not into expectations about a future driven mostly by anxiety and fear.

Our body-brain system is designed to provide what is needed in one form or another. It has a code for wellness. It does not lie nor create self deception - unless something interferes. And there the problems begin. The body signals go on continuously monitoring the "condition our condition is in," whether what we are doing is good for us or not so good, even harmful. Do we listen? Sometimes, mostly when things are just not going well, or we are desperate. The same system also allows for a self-image, an ego identity to form with all of its external demands, inhibitions, expectations, and conditionings to which we become attached and identified. And that is where the self-conflict starts to take off and grow and grow. After a while, we keep either pushing the body boundaries, by example, the "work harder" (not always smarter) driver which can be analyzed as *fear of never having enough* and always wanting more. (Is this the basis of the "American Dream" once a golden opportunity and now an anxiety about having it all?) There the stress grows: fear of failure, shame-guilt for not succeeding, and with it the internalization of anxiety. In this state it is difficult to experience equilibrium and more likely to gradually feel depressed. This vicious cycle feeds ever more stress and anxiety, a setup for body problems galore! While the phenomenon is universal, like a rampant disorder it can manifest virulently in some societies more than others.

Whenever the primary value is not the common good but rather ego-dominated personal aggrandizement we are much more susceptible to body disorders. When as a value *more is better* then fear of not having enough arises. The social fabric gets weakened as competitive endeavors become (in the words of the English political philosopher Thomas Hobbes) "a war of all against all". Two world wars demonstrated that. This time around we still do it, just less cataclysmic, selective and softer targeted, with cover-up.

Psycho-Somatic (Psycho-Physical) Pain Disorders

There are so many cases of pain disorders that have no identifiable, testable, medically scientific basis upon which a course of treatment or cure can be applied. But pain there is, and something is driving it. This in itself creates a stress of unknowing and with it an anxiety preoccupation in the patient who might be thinking: *"There must be something structurally wrong with me that no one has yet found."* The new driver of the problem then becomes worry and anxiety. The first thing for such people, and almost anybody, is to look for something that works to at least alleviate the distress. If enough cover-up remedies can be found, many people will look no further. If the parts are available, as in the case of a bad hip, the tendency to take the hip replacement as the solution may become greater than the more natural biological intelligence – that is finding ways to keep the hip joints intact. Hip joints, knee joints, shoulder joints, and yes, teeth, are designed to last for life. They are destroyed only with accidents, abnormal stresses, certain diseases and fairly rare congenital disorders. On the psychological side, a conflicted self-image can take us off course, wreaking confusion which becomes *somaticized* into certain postural states. If for example you are conditioned to believe there is something wrong with you, deficient, not good enough, or, in some religious upbringing, that your body is something totally separate from soul (a source of trouble, temptation, sinfulness) the *cns* retreats going into a suspended self-protective state waiting until new instructions arrive. If the same system can be shown how to reconnect with itself and move with ease, power, and flow, it will be restored.

A Clinical Case of Split Body-Mind

A client of noteworthy professional standing in the field of medicine and psychiatry came referred to me presenting a significant persisting lower back problem with periodic bouts of acute pain. The client was also engaged in a regimen of exercises ranging from intense bicycling to swimming, to using weights. As with many, his tendency was to do too much forceful exercise to the point where his body was compromised by overuse, urged on by the internalized exercise ideology of "no pain, no gain" and "try harder, do more".

This messaging soon becomes a cns wired-in habit. By its very nature of adaptability it tries to accommodate and adjust to whatever the input may be. In this way the habit of overuse can get attached to one's self image conditioning both and wiring them in - just neuro mechanisms at work! Whatever you practice becomes wrapped into a pattern. Myelin is myelin, gets laid down and wrapped this way by repetition, reinforced by the conviction (remember cognitive dissonance?) that this must be the best way to do things. Feedback signals to the contrary are then overridden. Not a big leap to see how a behavior can become programmed in the body-mind complex. In this instance, the habit also serves as a temporary relief, much like someone hooked on any drug or substance. What is most interesting is that the client was observant and aware enough to see that the hands-on and movement education applications I was messaging was producing positive effects: much reduced pain and more mobility. He knew it had value and could work.

Then at a point where he had to make the choice, he decided to discontinue. How come? Of course, the superficial excuses proffered are the usual, such as "no time... other commitments... too busy... my schedule is demanding," and so on. Later he revealed to his referring colleague a different story: "I know this method could help me, but not now. I might have to get worse before I am ready to get better."

The Limitations of Thinking Your Way Through

*T*hinking is a many sided brain function with many interpretations surrounding it. Being what it is, at times it leads to just as much ambivalence and confusion about choices as it does about clarity. When we are anxious, thinking degenerates into worrying about what ifs, a mental agitation that generates negative stress with unpleasant, unwholesome, even damaging effects. Psychosomatic disorders increase with unresolved stresses. Add to this *habituation*, also a positive-negative two-edged sword of our body-mind adaptation to the stresses of life, quickly turning from helpful servant to a compulsion and controller. (Recall the previous story of Harry and Harriet who began to realize that a new strategy to solve the problem of a flooding basement, rational and well thought through as it was, one that offered the best chance ever would also require a change in habits of adaptation.) Thinking one's way through any problem or situation at the *cerebral* level does not work if the initial process does not start with the older and deeper levels of the brain sometimes referred to as the primal-intuitive and the emotional limbic. The implication is this: all parts of the brain must be in sync to generate what I call true and more confident somatic thinking which by its very interconnected process turns ordinary thinking into discerning mind, one that can make choices without generating more ambivalence.

At first this may sound irrational but actually makes sense once we understand the phenomenon of the brain and *cognitive dissonance*. Getting out of pain despite worsening conditions or facing risky unpredictable surgical intervention is not enough to stop many people. Staying in a familiar zone that is somehow manageable takes precedence over the choice of changing horses in mid stream - even if it is a pain-prone stream. The internal dynamic of cognitive dissonance further explained goes something like this: to make a change - which might even be seen by the person to make total sense - comes up against the inertia of the existing and invested habit. To take a different path which might well resolve the problem might also be threatening, activating more anxiety and ambivalence. Better to follow the familiar even if it eventually ruins your body. The familiar is valued as the preferred course than the unfamiliar one. And of course this is how the presumably intelligent make unintelligent decisions and end up with unresolvable body problems, surgeries, and degeneration for the rest of their lives.

Where to Go from Here

As described in the previously cited case of Cora, there is a constant drama of muted sufferers who can "just live with it" and carry on but always feel the grip of the restricted life. Is this our fate? Is it inevitable, really necessary? Is there no exit, no escape, as many uninformed realists and religious doomsday predictors would have it? In this time of incredible technological accomplishments and the proliferation of everything from soup to nuts in the realm of therapy, exercise, health and extended longevity, the questions to ask are why is there such an increase in the instances of pain and disability and how to get out. There is no answer from inside the box. The only way is to take the road less seen or traveled when the signals indicate. Some of the findings of neuropsychology point the way.

Ambivalence and Psychosomatics

On first view ambivalence may seem normal, usual, no big deal. From a psycho-somatic point of view it looks and acts more like a state of confusion, conflicted interests and indecision. In the world of nature it is not so normal, and from the biological imperative where decision is needed on the spot ambivalence becomes more dysfunctional. Among human beings it is actually cultivated in many unconscious ways that most of us are not aware of, as in learned beliefs, behaviors, and social attitudes. Let's look at the central dynamic here: conflict within oneself. Ambivalence is often emotionally loaded, unlike deliberation which is just evaluation without heavy emotional charge. Conflicts within oneself, especially if they become habitual, create two voices at least each one representing part of the ego invested in that action, behavior or emotion. These ego states once formed now compete and grow into a symbiosis. More ambivalence, more ego. When we are in constant doubt or inner questioning we may be splitting ourselves, creating ego voices in the head talking to each other. What that also means at the psychosomatic level is that one cannot be fully into the present moment experience of sensing, feeling and moving. The mind becomes restless going back and forth among the choices as in which one is better, which one is to be avoided. There are feelings and somatic disturbances that go with it. These emotional agitations become programmed and now hard to get out of because every decision takes on one or more voices. No matter which side is considering, the other is agitating. Hard it is then to be fully into the experience, and so it keeps repeating. But does ambivalence just remain in some sectioned off psychological department of the brain? Nice way out but not the reality.

Change requires redirection and reconnection. There are ways out of ambivalence but they require dedicated commitment such as religious vows, constant group support, monitoring or ongoing psychotherapy, all of which are enormously time-energy consuming and not efficient. As we noted, Eastern practices involved the body: walking, doing yoga, martial arts, tai chi, and relaxing the mind through sitting meditation, mantras and chanting. Feldenkrais and others focused on body awareness through movement to reprogram the nervous system, bypassing old emotional reactions, mind wandering, indecision, and ambivalence. Better results do follow but still it is emotionally challenging to be fully and courageously (not recklessly) trusting one voice, one choice, what you're entering - being fully present. The new frontier being explored and developed is psycho-somatic integration through movement awareness exercises.

Releasing Emotional Energies

Psychology has a variety of means for releasing, redirecting, even reframing disruptive emotional energies or imbalances. But strangely, few work through the very pathway configurations and neural tissue components that drive the patterns of behavior. Medication (not prevention) is the prevalent form of treatment in Western cultures. Western psychology inherited a body-mind division going back centuries.

In acupuncture, as in Taoist practices, using meridians and points, emotional energy can be released and redirected. For example: release of anger is associated with the liver organ by doing certain physical or internal energizing movement actions connecting along contact points. The same energy can then be transformed (alchemized) into a positive emotive feeling state such as *kindness*.

In Emotional Freedom Technique (EFT), release of emotional tension can be induced through touch-tapping along specific pathway meridians. One of these important points is just below the collarbone at the juncture of the 2nd rib, if you know where that is. Makes sense neuro- somatically, not woo-woo at all. Opening the space between 2nd rib and clavicle allows for better fuller breathing, incompatible with anxiety, anger, or depression. Try it out.

Case of Affliction-Redemption

She came referred, with a history of severe jaw, neck and shoulder pain (already having had a jaw disc replacement that eventually failed). In her thirties, married with children, she regularly cringed all her life in a protective form of self-defense, her back curving, her shoulders tightening, her mid-spine stiffening against a constant barrage of verbal and psychological abuse. She was told she was no good by her mother - who constantly berated her - and was rejected when she found herself pregnant. Her father did nothing to protect her. By the time she came to see me she was on anti-anxiety depressants plus a number of other medications.

She responded to treatment, felt moments of "extraordinary relief," but never committed to the practice, never attended classes, did only a few exercises to get relief thereby neglecting the most important piece, taking full responsibility for self-care. Because of pain and other factors she tended to avoid dealing with her upper body and not doing the exercises she needed most. Beset by pain she tried a variety of different medications and some initial psychotherapy (which she resisted and denied as necessary). To deal with anxiety and depression she found meditation helpful, but it did not lead her out. I had given her the tools and stopped treating, but something was missing: the intention (kept from having its voice heard by what Tibetan Buddhist psychology calls the "demon" of the ego).

A few years later she reported she had had neck surgery that helped for a while. But soon the pains returned. They were exacerbated by a minor whiplash auto injury. MRI's showed nothing conclusive, but when we need to find a cause, we keep looking. Eventually a medical doctor told her the cause of her problem was "cervical compression." Still in denial she told me that her problems "had nothing to do with my posture, or exercise, or my mother. It was the cervical disc." What she could not, did not want to see was her own body posture of anxiety, her predisposition to position herself with head and neck craned forward. Shame and guilt can be major path blockers. Even ego pride is often a cover-up, a defense against anxiety. When we are emotionally fixated (in her case about age 15) the protection route is in not wanting to see. Behind the body pains - neck, jaw and all - was the now dead but internalized image of her guilt-imposing mother. The regrets that followed never led to a completed resolution pathway of self connection and deep relaxation. A self-image of abuse had taken deep roots, an she was not ready to relinquish it. "My poor dead mother! I need to always remember her. I feel so bad about it all..." In spite of this, Avida learned to be responsive and welcomed one truly functional beneficial practice: sitting *meditation, a path of centering. I helped her to be able to sit, breathe, be aligned and comfortable. This became her way of managing anxiety and maintaining a difficult but still viable life.*

[Postscript: The one demon she had not yet mastered is fear, resulting in her continuing dependency upon medical treatment. After many years, I heard from her sounding very depressed, "three shoulder operations, another on the jaw…" A case of failure, or a continuing process of self-discovery?]

If you then can redirect the feeling into an intentional choice of a better state of emotional equilibrium, you may be able to move away from continuous need for recovery and rehabilitation treatment. Most conventional as well as alternative therapies simply restore - if they succeed - the status quo ante, that is, the previous patterned condition before the condition generated problems. By example from the car analogy again: imagine for a moment you have a tire continuously losing pressure. So with constant attention you keep it going by putting in more air. Not as good as performing a repair. The problem keeps recurring, the superficial repair did not resolve the real cause behind both leak. If the problem is driven by body tissue tensing and self-conflicting mental-emotional reactions, this leads to more distress and disturbance.

What we often mean by emotional stress is a yes/no conflict in our bodies. One part is saying do this, the other do that. Since the *cns* does not allow saying yes and no at the same time what you have is a yes, negated by a no, recast again as a yes, and so on. This throws the *cns* rhythms out of sync. Pain responses are a normal consequence. The physical process counterpart would be something like this: doing exercise that you do not really want to do because it is part of an external then internalized demand, a fear-based motivation prescribed but not enjoyed. This alone can and often does generate stress resulting in pain, then rationalized into the familiar *no pain, no gain.* One learns to use pain as an indicator that something good lies in repeating it.

How Habits Get Internalized: Engram Fixation

Any psycho-emotional complex eventually becomes an *engram*, a total cerebral cortex memory, and by implication a neuromuscular habit built in deeply. Someone who has recurrent pain also learns ways to get out of the pain, at least for a while. This negative type of adaptive learning is not sustaining and eventually becomes dysfunctional. Consider all the escape from pain and discomfort mechanisms people use, from eating more, consuming more alcohol, more medications, recreational drugs, sleeping for long periods, and so on. Each repetition sets the pattern deeper. The system begins to identify ego with the adaptation, losing connection with one's original nature. There is also a consolation prize, a payoff, a trickle down, getting something out of it. The entire body pattern expresses the engram. Even the desire to change can now be internally resisted. Treatments that are based on forcing a change rarely succeed. The now addictive expectations need a transformation in intention and behavior, a different quality of somatic experience which then can be embodied.

What then is the relation to mental activities? When examined they appear to be extraordinarily complex, difficult to follow, and regarded as psychologically *chaotic from Taoist, Zen and Buddhist perspectives.* But after a while, and many studies, it turns out that the mind may well be operating on patterns that are following a different kind of process - seemingly unpredictable, inscrutable, unreadable - yet making sense from the somatic tracking view. One thing is still clear and compelling: anything that we feel, think or do in the mental or emotional sectors comes down through the same *final common pathway and is then* expressed in our posture, gestures, actions and behavior. As the body-mind system grows, develops, matures and functions well, so does our mental and emotional development match and resonate in sync. The worst outcomes are associated with blockages, constriction, restriction, poor body pathway organization and navigation. These are usually the result of psychophysical factors that have disrupted and confused the natural directional pathway mechanisms - like driving on a washed out road. Which came first, the physical or the mental, is similar to the often posed "chicken and egg" dilemma. Either end. It does not matter. The hang-up is only in how we perceive what is happening and how to manage it.

The following clinical stories illustrate various aspects of the psychosomatic process and the challenges each person met.

Case of Retarded Recovery and Somatic Amnesia

A once very athletic woman in her 50's, former basketball player and now a college team coach had a serious auto accident resulting in a broken shoulder kept immobilized for several months. During the long recovery she noticed something was wrong, not so much with her shoulder but in the non-impacted lower body seriously affecting her walking gait. She could obtain no medical explanation. Over a period of three years, trying out all the known and applied therapies available (in a fairly medically prolific and advanced area), still no progress. How can this be?

Whenever on her feet standing or walking she was in pain. Both hips were almost frozen, stiffened, and her gait awkward. She had regressed to a basic right to left shuffle. After two sessions of CMI relearning treatment she already felt a major difference. She reported reduced pain and hope about improvement "for the first time in years." I had begun by first relieving overworked muscles that were now substituting for the weakened and stressed once primary efficient hip joint movements. That is after all what those muscles must do in such conditions. The cns recruits and directs another group of muscles and fascia to take over for a lost function - DNA instructions at work. But these muscles and joints also have to work more and get no relief. At some point they shorten, losing lengthening and eventually go into lock down, or worse, painful spasm.

What was the process to get her brain to recognize and somatically think its way out of this vicious cycle. What did I need to see or do to connect with her brain-cns system to access new signals from within?

First I had to help install an external body mapping software she could use but never had. This provided a grounding, a foundation, a way of following a direction out of debilitation. Otherwise it's treatment dependency for life, and not likely sustainable. Because of her training in sports and exercise, this approach made sense. Coaches think in terms of strategies! She was receptive. A science-fact based approach had more appeal than some of the more mysterious (woo-woo) alternatives. In basketball and other sports the players have to think strategy, using play patterns that involve working together. This served then as the frame in which I could map her movements using her own body pathways the brain/cns would recognize.

There was still another side: the psycho-physical part of the process. Pain was the great motivator. When powerful levering joints do not move efficiently the muscles must work harder. But working harder is stressful, unpleasant, a slow degeneration road, in conflict with body's nature which in all creatures seeks efficiency and relaxation. Realizing this ingrained habit she was receptive and soon discovered (through an awareness tracking exercise) a prior "shadow," a predisposing lifestyle habit of always pushing herself too much, overworking and tensing up, feeling insecure. It was no longer just the accident but the path back to recovery that was both physically and psychosomatically blocked, with spine and other joints greatly reduced in mobility. None of her treating therapists had been able to see this complexity of background with hidden factors. No one had been able to explain her pelvis seizing up, the back pains, the loss of functional gait. At this point she was becoming both more aware and empowered.

She had drifted into what one well-known body practitioner and writer called "somatic amnesia" [Thomas Hanna described this condition as one of forgetting or losing connections. It is particularly a syndrome with people who live " in their heads," separated from body feelings and feedback.] I also refer to this condition as a psychosomatic disconnect.

As soon as these parts of herself were reconnected and reintegrated she responded. The joints began to move allowing her to walk with less pain. The missing pieces, the hidden shadowed parts needed to be brought out, reconnected and redirected. How else to explain lack of recovery especially in athletic people who respond to injuries faster than most. In previous years athletic, able to run, play sports, do exercise, and now unable to even walk without always being in pain? What happened between points A and B? An accident that one does not recover from indicates lost connections. Again, most therapeutic treatments and medical exams do not address these issues.

In this case the predisposing pattern of muscle and joint tightness was always there, covered up with forceful movements and exercises which at least stimulated blood circulation and helped discharge accumulated tissue toxins. The accident halted all of this. Now she was taking the path less traveled and on to a new way. Signs of improvement were evident as she slowly began to walk and feel better. However, the severe wearing of the hip joints that had taken place over the years now became the impasse that would greatly limit further progress. For one of the few times in my professional career I supported an orthopedic physician's clear documentation and demonstration that the parts were simply worn out and beyond regeneration. At first very reluctant, she now made the decision to undergo hip replacement as the next step - a decision indicating courage and trust in her own ability to improve and do the activities she enjoys following years of somatic anxiety and near depression. It worked!

Case of Fear of "Falling Apart"- A Doomsday Scenario Reversed

Regeneration vs the Slow Degeneration process

He came to me presenting a long history of problems, pain, with medical interventions and surgeries that only worsened his condition-all expressed in significant movement restrictions, especially walking and swimming. He was at that time unable to go down to the floor and come up again without using a chair. Once very athletic, a fast runner and distance-hitting golfer, now reduced to living with a pain-body, a constant feeling of tightness and limited mobility. A medical procedure for a condition of hernia, followed by a number of badly executed alternative therapy interventions, left him in more pain and immobility. M. was dependent now on constant treatments, from scar tissue to weekly massage to anything else that might help him just move without feeling totally trapped in a tightened and tormented body accompanied by the shadow fear that his body might fall apart at any time.

But as he learned to apply the method, and retrain his brain-body nervous system by following the core movement lesson-exercises I devised for him, he was on a regeneration path, eventually even able to run again. Getting up and down is no problem any longer. The progress continues with marked improvement, now walking up to 4 miles and playing golf fairly well for the *first time in years. How did this turnaround take place? What is regeneration all about? Can anyone experience it? Are we dealing with a unique situation, easily dismissed by the medical profession as an anomaly, or are we touching into something more fundamental, like tuning into the body's capacity to heal and improve by following specific movement exercises based on efficient body pathways. In essence, listening to our signals from within.*

Case of Feeling "Hopeless"

He came with a back, hip, and recurring knee problems. Within five sessions he seemed to feel recovered and able to continue on his own. As a professional psychologist sitting all day, his main and only reliable exercise was walking almost daily. The problem however was not resolved. It was clear to me that his lower back and hip imbalances would likely flair up again. A year later he again contacted me, this time in recovery from a meniscus knee operation (his second), and not able to walk several months after the arthroscopic surgery without acute pain. Now he was desperate, depressed, and determined to stay with the process this time around. However, the biggest obstacle in the process proved to be the psychophysical factor. N. seemed to both know himself and yet not know anything about how his body moved. It is as if he unconsciously avoided knowing anything more than what was needed to get him up, down and around. He could not follow simple instructions or read his own body's innate established movement patterns. Despite his talents and abilities professionally, it was as if his body was foreign to him, a rented instrument not his own, once outside the realm of familiar imprinted movement habits. With each session he would feel better, then at home doing easy recommended exercises he would go into a kind of depressive panic.

Finally in session he declared: "I just can't learn this... I'm hopeless... Too old... Can't get it... I'll just live with a knee brace and low back support, and keep going..." (sounding as if there might be an unconscious messaging like: "until I fall apart totally.")

At that point, my perceptive practitioner colleague who was attending the session intervened, and offered a change of approach: "Since you are here and I came in for the first time, and since you have paid for the session, would you be open to just lying down and letting me introduce a few things I see that might help?"

We in effect switched his attention away from the flair up emotional crisis (distraction technique) to an approach he could relate to in his own profession as a psychologist. This shift activated his curiosity though he still held back, cautiously passive, non-engaged. Now the two of us working in sync gradually introduced him to his own body muscles and joints in a non-threatening way, making small non-demanding invitations to feel connections. Still he did not really feel new sensory-motor happenings in his body until the circumstances were lined up right. At some point the shift was observable: he started to connect! On our part, by using this safe, non-confusing mode, by pointing out only what he could either observe or sense, he was not compromised in his self image of being hopeless. Together we were able to manually trigger different responses as his held muscles released their contractions and joints began moving in sync - a state in which pain is in effect alleviated. He got up, walked and experienced no acute pains, to the point where he insisted on practicing the moves of walking as if now intent on learning these so he would not just forget and get depressed. [Then he went on an extended vacation. No follow up has occurred.]

Chapter 8
Varieties of Movement Maintenance: Comparisons and Contrasts

By now, one observation has emerged conclusively: life without the right ways of movement and exercise will be compromised. And this by all known statistical and research evidence bears out in various forms, shapes, and styles the world over, from prehistoric to primitive and modern.

Running

"Wired to Run, and Think-Evolving the ability to run may also have made our ancestors smarter, suggesting that exercise can be healthy for the brain as well as the body...As the forests of Africa gave way to the plains, our ancestors came down out of the trees and started to run. Ancient humans chased down larger prey by working together in sophisticated hunting groups that could follow prey for hours before actually seeing it, using clues to track the animals and infer their movements. In order to run such long distances, hominins grew taller and stronger, developing long legs and tendons, wide shoulders, and weight-bearing joints. This aerobic capacity was unprecedented among primates."

-Hayley Dunning, <u>The Scientist</u>, July 26, 2012

"Running was the most popular type of exercise (ages 22-45) followed by lifting weights and biking/hiking/outdoor activities." [according to a survey by the watch company Timex]

Running was also my prevalent form of exercise for years and seemingly worthy of a longer discussion than I am offering here. The many books that have been written about running describe more about the romanticized than the actual side. Even though it offers substantial benefits such as cardio, it is paradoxically the one activity related to the most injuries. Some 80% of runners as I have noted from several reports have and will likely continue to have injuries that will seriously compromise their ability to run. I am one of them.

What then is the main driver behind the running craze? Is it really an enjoyable activity? Can it be sustained for a lifetime, like walking, tai chi, even golf? Is it truly then a functional activity of daily life? The answer is: *clearly not.*

Running is done the world over but only by the young, and most often for practical reasons like getting somewhere, hunting, or as in sports. Beyond a certain age, unless occasionally done as part of activities of daily life, running can become dysfunctional. I not only ran from age 24 to age 60, but frequently engaged in road races. The final result was to severely tear my knee meniscus - the most common injury of runners - effectively ended my running. From that time on, I then took up fast walking, race walking (which could also cause injuries and in my case could not be sustained), and eventually to more trekking, the most sustainable and healthiest of them all.

Exercise - Gym Style

The gym environment is one form of an exercise setup with a wide assortment of equipment made available. It offers several options for those who prefer or need this kind of dependable, quasi-social and physically stimulating ambience. Some of the equipment in the form of strength exercise machines are impressively specific and efficient in their mechanics, allowing focus on body sectors and isolating groups of muscles. Motion-oriented aerobic equipment such as treadmills, step-stair, ski and rowing machines, ellipticals, stationary bikes can be impressive, developing muscles and offering the user a better body image. The modern gym is a unique modernized and transmogrified form of our ancient Western ancestry, the sports palladiums of Greece and Rome.

The gym may also offer a variety of more total body movement exercise including yoga, aerobics, spinning, many styles of strength training, various styles of martial arts, Pilates, Nia, Zumba, kick boxing, and many other related quick-do, fast pace forms. It all can help, looks good on the surface - and yet something makes me hesitate to regard this style of self-care as beneficial and sustainable long term. Here are my concerns:

- The tendency to emphasize isolation far more than integration
- The emphasis on muscle development - looking good - rather than on the far more substantial biomechanical basis using body levers.
- The tendency towards forced exercises, push-pull efforting, the mindset of driven-ness, working harder, not smarter.

Check out the facial expressions of many gym-goers, often indicating more straining than natural pleasurable pursuit.

The gym also can become a place for the "gym rat", a now common expression describing those who make it an extension of home, the modern *homo sap* who keeps going and going, driven by the strange but understandable yet potentially dangerous hypnotically-inducing belief in "no pain, no gain". Unless that edge of pain is felt, the belief is that nothing beneficial can possibly be happening.

Lastly, there is the temptation using weights to increasingly raise the threshold and lift more. This further programs and internalizes the message "to prove yourself, do the reps" - until pain sets in. Living with pain has become common, acceptable, and normalized. Why pain and achiness? Because the gym is not a set and setting to cultivate resonant movement flow nor more natural ways of integrating. Rather it is something closer to a sports complex where athletes push harder, do more sit-ups, get to feel, even execute, a brief period of performance-high. After, as the discomforts set in and the joints are strained, they then may likely settle down to a more sedentary lifestyle, usually gaining weight and becoming stiff in the joints - arthritis bound!

Not my first choice! Yes, from time to time I also indulge especially in seasonal weather conditions. I would go for that needed exercise and cardio tune up, a good pool swim where available, and always returning to the basics, the secret of the animals. They lift not, nor do they overstrain themselves on machines; nor do they do the "crunches", those muscle shortening sit-ups which can compromise joints and posture. But the animals are strong, flexible, fast, and far less plagued by arthritis! How can this be and what does it tell us? The same story that has been the theme song of this book.

Why not just carry around a fitness band and do many hundreds of exercises each day during breaks. Exercise as you sit. Add in a few miles of walking and you will likely get even more than the few hours a week at the gym (which may readily be sacrificed to other daily life concerns calling out). This becomes enjoyable even relaxing activity without the strain, the weight lifting, the grimacing face, the painful expressions. Still, don't throw out the baby with the bathwater! The gym can sometimes be the right place to go, right time and situation.

Dance as Expressive Exercise

The world of dance is vast. There is no tribe or culture which does not dance. It is also closely related in those tribal contexts with activities of daily life. Practiced just as an enjoyable movement it can do wonders for your body and longevity. Upgrade it to the level of an exercise it qualifies up there with the best. But the dancing I am referring to is not just the demanding, often forced, highly stylized form such as ballet, or even the many modern varieties from hip-hop on. It is more like popular dance forms which can be done for a lifetime. Almost all known ethnic and tribal people dance regularly as part of their village life style, and not just in special settings. Many African and Native American tribes danced before going into some dramatic adventure, encounter, even battle, like the Zulus of South Africa who would run long distances, then dance, before fighting. Was it emotional release, energy activation, last minute social sharing, sexual stimulation, farewell parting or even partying? The key in dance movements is to enter into a flow zone, physical entry, then into aesthetic, social and spiritual expression.

Yoga: Positive and Healthy, But Not Without Pitfalls

The appeal of yoga is still growing in the West and getting close to peaking. In the East it has diminished. What makes it appealing to westerners? Is it safe for most people? I have already alluded to my experience of yoga and still consider it the first of my transformative experiences. From a physiological and even biomechanical perspective, it has many sound features. The postures or *asanas* are expressive body-energy forms, the manifestations of connecting internally - in yoga parlance - to body, mind and spirit. Yoga has the power of a tested, tried and true tradition behind it. People beginning the practice, have a sense of being in something known, respected, able to be learned under the guidance of a knowledgeable teacher. What we now have more of is a demand and market for fast track training of then to become "certified" teachers.

What is also happening is the proliferation of many more neo-varieties of yoga than ever before, hardly time-tested and less controlled in quality, preparation and monitoring. With quasi-regulated training, many teachers are not fully developed, not taught in the biomechanical essentials, nor well prepared in body movement basics, nor adequate to the task of noticing and monitoring their students. The risk factors have been on the rise, and "yoga injuries" are now frequently discussed even in the yoga magazines.

The *asanas*, or postures, are body movement combinations designed or believed to produce certain effects, especially internally on glands and organs but only occasionally subject to scientific testing and validation. However, pragmatic results do count. The yoga student, like the consumer, needs to be better informed, more aware and self-guided (caveat emptor!).

My main concerns: while many elements of the old tradition still remain as part of yoga practice, the reality is that yoga has also become popularized into just another form of exercise, now multiplied into myriad schools. There is even a "yoga therapy," a kind of manual application often with overstretching - a yet another purported fix to body problems such as back pain, tension, and a host of current complaints brought on by our life style. Still hard to go wrong if the yoga style of your choice produces benefits.

Another of my concern is about knowing what you are doing. It is true that myofascial lengthening needs to occur before stretching and strengthening can be effective. But in many yoga practices the emphasis has been by tradition largely on the stretching component and then with strengthening. In earlier times and in a less busy, consumer driven culture such as India, more time was allowed for slow stretching. Time constraint was not the issue as it is today. Stretching done too quickly creates as we noted, a muscle spindle, elastic band-like reaction. As the nervous system detects a muscle being taken beyond its normal resting state of tonus, it experiences such a stretch as abnormal, initiating a contractile physiological reaction usually felt later as pain. Under such conditions the benefit is greatly diminished, if not negated entirely.

The attraction of quick stretching is that it tends to produce an immediate effect in the form of stimulated blood flow, a sense of relaxation in some instances more like a tranquillizer than an awakener into awareness. In fact, the real awareness may actually be dulled. Over-stretching might be compared to taking an alcoholic drink. It feels good and warm on the intake, but later has disturbing side effects. Yoga injuries from improper stretching have now become a popularly recognized category of concern, with many articles written on this subject.

On the plus side, yoga done slowly has beneficial features. The practice evokes awareness and relaxation responses. It also lengthens, stretches and strengthens. It focuses the mind through the body/central nervous system. It tends more towards awakening the brain rather than putting it to sleep while producing desirable endorphins, and at least potentially more somatic awareness.

From a bio-functional movement perspective, yoga may not be nearly as effective or able to be continued for a lifetime, as for example Tai Chi Qigong or walking (I've noticed over forty years of practice as a therapist and yoga instructor how many people have discontinued because of difficulties and injuries). On the positive side, yoga can be beneficial as prep exercises in walking, running, playing soccer, and even as now used in the hard sports like football. Yoga postures, though often extreme make some sense structurally and can be explained in biomechanical terms using body pathway mapping.

There are known and testable physiological effects of yoga especially with the emphasis on slow stretching while breathing and relaxing. There are also psychophysical benefits of yoga such as controlling the wandering quirky, erratic human mind by inducing relaxation, calmness and centering. Yoga is in the tradition of disciplines promoting self-knowing through body-centered practice. That was the project and the design of its first great mapper and compiler, Patanjali (circa 800 BC).

Yoga: The View From Physics, Biomechanics and Physiology

As a body-mind system of exercise and meditation, yoga uses an energy map [*prana*] centering on the spine and moving up through centers called *chakras,* and postural positional movements called *asanas.* But posture as such is not recognized in the central nervous system which is primarily oriented around detecting changes in functional position. *Posture* in real terms is dynamic not just static. Movement counts more than staying still. It represents our self-image, our state of being, our responsiveness and how we organize ourselves. Yoga *asanas* are done in the same field of gravity as are all movement actions, requiring a sense of balance, position, and direction of movement even if apparently static. They follow and express some root bio-physical principles. If we perform with felt understanding and awareness of these root movement components the results will be positive. If they are forced, the results will be mixed, compromised, stressful to joints and tendons. The best and most sensible guideline, the one least likely to produce any discomfort or pain, is simply this: lengthen before stretching, and maintain the sensory-motor feel of resonance in the postures. Basic bone, joint, muscle-connective tissue physiology applies to all people and the movement practices they do. For muscles to work well, and for the benefits to be maximized, these are the conditions needed:

- **Joints** must move without friction or turbulence.

- **Muscles** must lengthen in order to produce the force (energy) to contract and work functionally [called the *resting potential*].

- **Connective tissue** (the fascia) must spread and maintain "tensegrity" with the direction of the lengthening and elongation.

Somatic Synergy is the interaction of bones, joints, muscle, fascia, plus mindset and affect. It works best when we are in resonant motion flow. [See our DVD *Yoga Using Core Movement Pathways.* The CMI system of mapping shows how the body transmits all forces along primary pathways, which link into secondary ones.]

Movement done slowly with awareness of the feel changes the experience. This way of stretching is not likely to activate a muscle spindle reaction. The nervous system can accept the stretch as part of the lengthening movement sequence. Done in this way, yoga offers a way of developing awareness and stimulating neuro-somatic relearning.

Tai Chi Qigong

Of all the known exercise systems in the world, qigong is the oldest, going back some 4000 years to early China. It is the one system which is closest to even what we know today about how energy moves in the body. In addition, it is a unified system, part of Taoist body, mind and spirit practices, and linked closely with oriental medicine.

What makes it unique is that all of the movements were derived by studying the ways of animals and nature. These early practitioners had only an intuitive but pragmatic understanding of how gravity and energy (forces) moved in the body. The concept of *meridians,* or pathways conducting life sustaining and healing energies, and the time-tested practical semi-science that emerged from it appears to me to be by far the most advanced, extending to the present resurgence.

Acupuncture which is based on meridian energy flow, has become widely accepted even in the medical world. But the root of acupuncture came out of the qigong practices, the mainstay of health and longevity for centuries. Qigong exercises were in effect self-applied meridian stimulants and can be seen to follow the same primary six core movement pathways that we discovered and mapped - a simple reminder that all human movement has a common basis and a common origin. With the spread of this practice into the entire Western culture we see some of the same adaptive tendencies as with yoga, such as teachers making students forcefully hold positions for too long. Many who have not learned nor been taught the real physics-based body alignment end up having problems especially with the knees, and cannot continue. As a practitioner and certified teacher of tai chi qigong for many years, I have often witnessed this phenomenon and worked with numerous students having problems as a consequence. Performing these practices in the right way can benefit you for a lifetime, like walking until the day we say goodbye!

[See our CMI DVD: **Tai Chi Qigong Using Core Movement Pathways, 2015**]

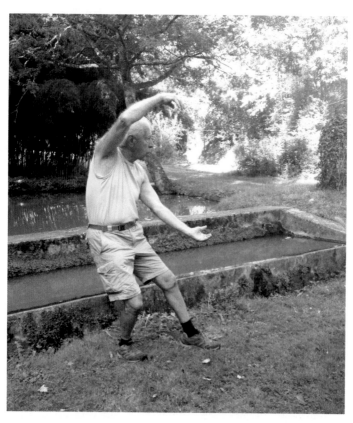

Chapter 9
Needed Changes in Traditional Hands-On Therapies

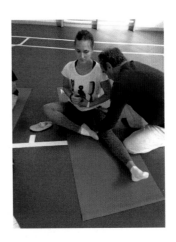

Besides the most known conventional therapies such as physical therapy, chiropractic, massage, acupuncture, a growing number of alternative bodywork modalities have emerged, each with its own approach. Most are based on offering some form of treatment, relief of pain, prevention or rehabilitation including accompanying benefits such as evoking relaxation responses or stimulating body systems. Even though validating research and results may be still lacking, or in question, still in one form or another these will likely continue. The central challenge of our times is to help develop and emerge systems of therapeutic education which can and will improve the body's ability to stay well and fit for the duration of life.

Conventional therapies often remain limited to only temporary results including improvements. In sports and rehabilitation applications these therapies can contribute to a certain amount of necessary maintenance. Massage, chiropractic and acupuncture plus several of the new emergent alternative therapies are mostly passive modes of treatment. What is often lacking - and now known through somatic neuroscience - is sufficient central nervous system (*cns*) stimulation called *neurogenesis*. Introducing movement has a double advantage: it benefits both the practitioner and the client. As neuroscience advances, it keeps revealing that movement is the major factor in activating learning and improving the brain. Movement done well improves all body functions and stimulates new neural pathways. Several recently publicized studies reveal that as little as 15 minutes of any cardio-active motion will produce more circulation than any amount of passive manipulation. Adding the movement component to massage or chiropractic can lead to a significant enhancement the benefits. My own practice as well as those who I have trained in this approach corroborates this.

Maintenance and Regeneration: Related but Different

As therapists become more interested and educated in neuro-somatic hands-on applications they must challenge their own fixed and limiting habits and learn how to read the body and expand their hands-on skills to include both movement and neural circuitry stimulation, the gateway to *regeneration* itself. No matter how light or how deep the therapist applies manual force or pressure; no matter how long the practitioner works on the client, passive application can only achieve a certain amount of beneficial effects such as tissue stimulation, lymph drainage, myofascial release, and relaxation. There comes a point of no further gain. As with all mechanical and biomechanical systems, maintenance can at best only slow down degeneration. When movement is added and becomes integrated with functional exercise, it will inevitably lead to greater benefits. All this suggests that we need to encourage more active movement not only in our clients but also in ourselves.

If new learning is to come in there must be receptivity to the perspectives and contributions of other modalities. Like a university which houses disciplines of many kinds, so will these new approaches be acknowledged and supported.

Core Movement Integration (CMI) practitioners, each and often with their own training backgrounds learn to read movement pathways through both hands-on stimulation, guidance, connectivity, and lesson-exercises requiring implementation and practice. CMI trained therapists learn specific manual applications based on a commonly shared knowledge foundation, a common protocol, a sense of collaboration and integration with other somatic modalities. CMI body learning therapy begins with *somatic empathy*, tuning in to the client's patterns without imposing, listening in by touch to client's movement pathway rhythms. This approach can be applied to all forms of manual therapy from medically to energy based.

Skills and Tools

CMI practitioners draw from several sources including and going beyond original training foundations. The key is to stimulate awareness in the client by means of somatic-empathic touch and movement pathway sensory motor connections

We use them in the following ways:

- Simply observe the patterns of movement in the body system. Make hands-on contact and follow without directing, instructing, criticizing or imposing. Be there with the person. Listen in.

- As client receptivity permits gently introduce a pathway pattern. Observe how and when the client accepts the moves, the clarification, differentiation, or redirection.

- Observe tissue restrictions which with appropriate skills can usually be released along the path without force. The purpose is to invite receptivity not resistance.

- Once the person's nervous system is more relaxed and receptive, pathway direction and resonant motion flow can be suggested, induced, or assisted.

One CMI practitioner, Arthur Madore, LMT, defines *empathic touch* as "manual contact that duplicates the state of being of a body segment . . . the quality of the hand melting and merging into the body. There is an exact duplication of the speed and direction of a movement without imposing any agenda." This is also fundamental in the hands-on work of Feldenkrais called *functional integration* (FI). It communicates rapport, understanding and safety.

CMI practitioners apply what they know, from *myofascial release* techniques to *positional release technique* [Denise Deig, PT], and *counterstrain* to quickly release connective tissue restrictions for smoother movement function. A shortening of the fascia can prevent full, comfortable *range of motion* [ROM] both actively and passively. This can be addressed through repetitive lesson-exercises using an awareness through movement process brought to the point of stretch, or through specific myofascial release techniques. Where reorganization of fascia was a primary goal of Rolfing, reorganization of the pattern of movement is the goal of both CMI and Feldenkrais.

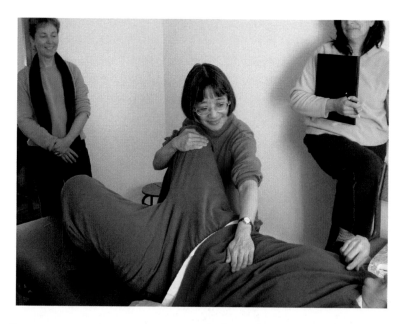

Intention is key - a recognizable and somatically demonstrable clear path of choice with its emotional and physical movement expression. Intention is a unifying state of being containing a relaxation response, fuller breathing, relaxed muscles, lighter facial expression - a preferred condition.

Enhancing Somatic Awareness

Touch applied in the right place can have a powerful sensory-motor effect. CMI hands-on work can enhance brain recognition, a remembering of bio-physical movement pathways. It can greatly facilitate safe and secure learning, opening a new window of perception. This process does not stop here. *Unless followed up by self-initiated essential exercises - gentle, small, larger, or stronger - according to the person's ability and intention to receive and utilize them, the myelinization learning and wrapping process does not take place.*

Summary

The sheer number of emergent bodywork and healing modalities presents a polarizing tendency: stick with the familiar or move into creative change solutions. Many of them, like researchers seeking to find a better medication or treatment technology, miss the opportunity to address the source of the problems.

Core Movement Integration is a risk-taking method but with a solid foundation in biomechanics, physiology, and neuroscience. We are creative change-agents with underfunded, limited but convincing clinical testing that offer an integrated self-care approach which can resolve body problems and improve the human condition. We have developed a comprehensive exercise and core-strengthening program that can both prevent, maintain and improve our now precarious extended but debilitating life conditions.

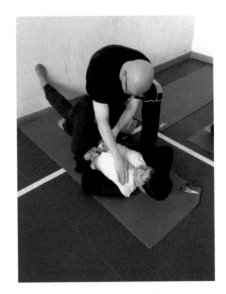

Bibliography

Coyle, Daniel. *The Talent Code.* Arrow Books, 2010.

Davidovits, Paul. *Physics In Biology and Medicine.* Elsevier Inc., 2013. 4th edition

DellaGrotte, J. *Instructions From Within: Core Integration.* CI Training Institute, Inc., 2007.

Feldenkrais, Moshe. *Body & Mature Behavior.* International Universities Press, 1981.

Feldenkrais, Moshe. *The Potent Self: A Guide to Spontaneity.* Harper & Row, 1985.

Hanna, Thomas. *Somatics: Reawakening the Mind's Control of Movement, Flexibility and Health.* Addison-Wesley, 1988.

Lodge, Henry and Christopher Crowley. *Younger Next Year.* Workman Publishing Company, Inc., 2007.

Pert, Candace B. *Molecules of Emotions: The Science Behind Mind-Body Medicine.* Touchstone, 1999.

Ratey, John. *Spark: The Revolutionary Science of Exercise and the Brain.* Little, Brown and Company, 2008.

Rolf, Ida P. *Structural Integration: Gravity An Unexplored Factor in a More Human Use of Human Beings.* Boulder: The Guild for Structural Integration, 1963.

Yanker, G. and Burton, K. *Walking Medicine: The Lifetime Guide to Preventive & Therapeutic ExerciseWalking Programs.* McGraw-Hill, 1990.

DellaGrotte, Josef. "Going with the flow: Examining back pain syndromes as core postural weakness." *Physical Therapy-Advance* April 2005: 49-51.

DellaGrotte, Josef. "From Maintenance to Movement." *Massage Magazine* June, 2014.

Made in the USA
Columbia, SC
31 January 2020